ASPE
THE ELU

An Applied Rehabilitation Guide for Adults

Dedicated to Oded Eran, of blessed memory,
my soul mate, my love;
and to our children and grandchildren,
Miracles of creation.

Producer & International Distributor
eBookPro Publishing
www.ebook-pro.com

ASPERGER'S (ASD) THE ELUSIVE SYNDROME
An Applied Rehabilitation Guide for Adults
Benjamina Eran

Translation from the Hebrew: Ziona Sasson
Contact: oberan@mcc.org.il

ISBN 9781686095870

ASPERGER'S (ASD)
THE ELUSIVE SYNDROME

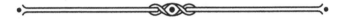

An Applied Rehabilitation Guide for Adults

BENJAMINA ERAN

CONTENTS

ACKNOWLEDGMENTS

With deepest gratitude and appreciation to all my colleagues who escorted me along my professional path and whose wisdom rings forth from the pages of this book:

Hava Baruch – Clinical Psychologist

Tova Averbuch – Social-Worker and Organizational Consultant

Professor Ofer Golan – Bar-Ilan University

Dr. Hila Mantin – Clinical Psychologist

Dr. Lior Friedman – Clinical Psychologist

My beloved daughter, Edna Eran, the treasure of my insights.

Last but not least, my many students in the training courses for group facilitators, whom I taught and with whom I grew.

*"I will give far more for the ability to get along with people than for any other ability."—**John D. Rockefeller***

PREFACE

NEED AS A SEARCH ENGINE

My 32-year-old daughter turned to me one day, surprised, and told me she had read on the internet about a phenomenon called "Asperger's,"[1] then added, "it's just like me." This discovery enabled us to understand the social hardships of adults who find it difficult to integrate socially, and triggered our journey in search of the most suitable help.

Following after my daughter's social development was a tricky journey. She was an intelligent and creative girl, who yearned to fit in with her peer group, and experienced exclusion and loneliness. As time passed, these difficulties increased, as did a growing distance away from her peer group, and loneliness played an increasingly greater part in her world.

---

1   In 2013, in the diagnostic manual DSM-5, the term "Asperger" was replaced by autism spectrum disorder (ASD). To remove all doubt, it is here noted that the term "Asperger" (ASD) is used throughout this book, as the population represented herein was defined as having "Asperger syndrome." This definition took root amongst the diagnosed clients, therapists, educators, families and the interested general public. The term "neurotypical" (NT) represents the variety of populations that are not on the autism spectrum (ASD). [Use of the male gender throughout the book represents both genders with absolute equality].

As my interest in Asperger's (ASD) deepened, I realized that research was at its height and that experiments were under way to develop and apply unique treatment programs. As a result, I decided to draw on my professional specialization in relevant areas and develop a rehabilitation program for adults with the syndrome.

The aim of this book is to help adults who are on the high-functioning autistic spectrum. It is meant to address the special needs of the adult population that suffers from social isolation and **its consequences**, whose members have the potential for their own individual development and the ability to contribute to society.

INTRODUCTION

A REHABILITATION PROGRAM FOR ADULTS WITH ASPERGER'S (ASD)

NEED GIVES RISE TO A RESPONSE

The thought that neurotypical people maintain meaningful communication naturally causes those diagnosed with Asperger's (ASD) – to feel incomplete and confused Willey (2000). In her book about Asperger's (ASD) in the family, Willey addresses those factors that drive people who suffer from the syndrome to escape and refrain from social contact. In their attempt to calm her before a social encounter, her close friends tell her that she should just act naturally. Her reaction is that this only works for those who have never experienced being mocked or laughed at because of **social mistakes,** and have never suffered shame because of their exaggerated efforts to please. Her insightful observation sheds light on the communication between people with Asperger's (ASD) and neurotypical people, a situation in which misunderstandings often develop that may lead to additional misunderstandings. In this situation, a person with the syndrome may feel lost and be preoccupied with searching for a safe haven, in order to feel focused and stable and avoid the anxiety caused by the interpersonal encounter. This is due to the many emotional scars he carries from experiences fraught with mockery and rejection in his childhood.

Adults with Asperger's (ASD) experience the world in a different way. They perceive it as a maze. Their difficulty is in navigating their way in a world they are unable to understand. Every frustration, anxiety and fear propels them toward seeking out shelter in familiar surroundings, in which they can fulfill their need for repetitiveness, routine and structuring their order of things. A sense of control helps them organize, sharpen and focus their functioning. This reality impacts on the quality of life of these adults, whom the surrounding environment perceives as incomprehensible and as people who don't know how to protect themselves.

They need help in developing social skills in order to enrich their survival tool kit. Asperger's (ASD) is not a "handicap," a term that conceptualizes helplessness, weakness, lack of ability and uselessness. On the contrary, people with Asperger's (ASD) have a great variety of capabilities: to learn, to grow, to cope and progress. They are able to show interest in another person's words and in his life.

Willey (2000) claims that if the neurotypical environment refrains from being **judgmental** toward adults with the syndrome, and accepts them as being differently unique, they will then be able to concentrate on what is essential for their existence and development.

It is possible to help adults with Asperger's (ASD) to connect to the neurotypical world, in keeping with their abilities, without losing touch with who they really are and what they need. The practical application is a rational and logical intervention via a rehabilitation program, based on a humanistic approach, professional knowhow, understanding and empathy of their existential experience, along with encouragement to fulfill their unique skills and potential.

The general intervention strategies should include practical and technical instructions for behavior management, methods of emotional support and activities for cultivating and developing social fitness, while taking into consideration the strengths and weaknesses of each and every individual.

An important component in the intervention program for people with Asperger's (ASD) is the need to reinforce their capacity for social and communicative coping. It addresses their reality, in which most of them are not lonely by choice, and tend to develop, toward adolescence, anxiety and depression. Therefore, it is essential and of top priority to instill social and communication skills as an integral part of the program.

In summary, as Klin stated (Klin et al, 2000), in every training program of social communication skills, priority should be given to efforts in developing skills of both the individual and his peer group. A fuller realization of the individual's natural talents will promote attaining satisfaction in employment, independence and the general emotional welfare of adults with Asperger's (ASD).

PART I

ASPERGER'S (ASD) –
THE ELUSIVE SYNDROME
A GENERAL REVIEW

CHAPTER 1

ASPERGER'S (ASD) - AN ELUSIVE SYNDROME OF DEVELOPMENTAL DEFICIENCY

Asperger's Disorder (ASD) is a syndrome characterized by neurotypical cognitive ability, on the one hand, and difficulties in social adaptation, on the other hand. It is a neuro-biological, neuro-psychological and developmental syndrome. This disparity between interpersonal and social dysfunction and cognitive ability therefore creates an elusive picture.

The syndrome manifests, inter alia, via an impairment in deciphering social codes and "reading" the social map, thus impacting on all spheres of life. Lorna Wing, in her introduction to Attwood's book (2007) writes that people with Asperger's (ASD) perceive the world differently from everyone else. This often leads them to confrontations with the conventional thinking, feeling and behavior that characterizes the neuro-typical population." (Attwood, 2007)

They cannot change, but they need help in finding ways to adapt to the world as is, to enable them to utilize their unique skills constructively, thus achieving independence in their adulthood.

This book focuses on adults with Asperger's syndrome (ASD). Adults with this syndrome are usually very pleasant and interesting, yet they encounter difficulties in forming relationships with people in their vicinity and in maintaining friendships. Each and every one of them copes with the core symptoms, which are neuro-biological in origin, intertwined with his or her unique personality components. Beyond the core symptoms of the syndrome itself are secondary problems that impact on how each one functions.

One mother of an adult with the syndrome successfully expressed the misgivings experienced by parents of ASD children during their early childhood years, when the child demonstrates unusual behaviors alongside good understanding and cognitive skills. This mother recognized early on her son's problematic attention span and difficulty in understanding authority and rules, together with his ability to learn on his own. When her son was about four years old, the boy's mother identified his adaptive impairment and expressed concern and confusion due to his high cognitive thinking skills. And, truly, this little boy, who is now an adult, clearly demonstrated his skills from a very young age.

Like many other families, our hero's family members also experienced hardships and misgivings. They "groped their way in the dark," and had to cope with frustrations and with the child's difficulty in understanding social situations and behavior codes. Regarding the difficulties that intensified with the crisis of adolescence, the mother noticed his basic lack of understanding in perceiving each person's place and deciphering social cues, even at the most basic level, even when all that is needed is a smile or some minimal recognition of another person.

Neurotypical infants will choose to pay attention to social cues, which connect them to the flow of social communication. In this manner, a structure of attention to interpersonal give-and-take begins to develop. The ASD child does not show much interest in the social interactions that take place around him, which will lead to undesirable consequences in the course of his development (Klein et al., 2000).

Gradually, as one advances in age, there is a greater manifestation of the lack of social attention, impaired understanding of social status, difficulty in interpreting non-verbal expression, and perhaps clumsiness in how one conducts himself physically, methodically and socially.

Social interactions progressively break down due to the fundamental deficiency of Asperger's syndrome (identifying social codes, etc.), and thus opportunities to experience social relationships are lost. They are crucial to the formation of one's personality during a child's and adolescent's developmental process. It can be concluded, therefore, that a significant part of the hardships in later life originate from this congenital social deficiency. Repeated failures in social relationships during childhood impede the ability to develop relationships during later stages in life, leading to seclusion and loneliness. This state of affairs obstructs social experiences, which, as is known, are a basic precondition for learning social and interpersonal codes and acquiring interpersonal behavioral skills.

This reality impacts on problems in deficient functional management in different areas, and hinders efforts to achieve personal and interpersonal goals.

Dr. Yuren-Hagash, in her introduction to Attwood's book (2007), notes that the adolescents yearn to come out of their bubble. Some remain devoid of any social ties and wonder why this has happened to them.

Asperger's (ASD), being a congenital syndrome, does not disappear with the onset of adolescence. Nonetheless, adults with ASD can be helped in improving their social skills and developing skills in neurotypical behavior, via therapy and rehabilitation programs specially tailored to their needs.

CHAPTER 2

ASPERGER'S (ASD) AND DIFFICULTIES IN
COMMUNICATION BEYOND WORDS

Christopher, the hero of *The Curious Incident of the Dog in the Night-Time* (Mark Haddon, 2003), describes simply and clearly how he experiences the inability to process the non-verbal dimensions of communication. The character tells us that people confuse him with actions like raising an eyebrow or sitting in a certain way, and many complicated things that he has to think about in a short time. Molcho in his book, Everything About Body Language (1998), states that a person uses body language naturally throughout his life, without being aware of it. He says that we cannot refrain from using body language as a means of communication, as our body reacts spontaneously and cannot "pretend," the way we can with words. Body language facilitates closer relationships between people and provides perceptions about their feelings, intentions and thoughts, through listening and observation.

We can become more understandable to ourselves and to others if we pay closer attention to our own physical signals and that of others. Effective non-verbal communication includes interpreting bodily signals, since bodily expression reflects what is happening inside oneself. Verbal language in itself is the descriptive channel of messaging, whereas body language is the experiential channel for transmitting information in the communicative process. For example: sparkling eyes, a glowing face, 'his face got clouded', 'he lost face', 'covered his face with his hands', etc.

For those diagnosed with the syndrome there is some limitation to their communication skills that is derived from difficulty in absorbing non-verbal information. Additionally, they find it hard to cope with cause-and-effect relationships and understand contents that do not have direct and logical congruence between their various parts (humor, practical jokes, paradoxical expressions, similes, manipulations and generalizations). This is manifested in their inability to understand and map out the social environment and navigate it. This chapter emphasizes the importance of the non-verbal language of communication in its impact on the social restraints for people with Asperger's (ASD).

In order to maintain qualitative communication between people, integration is needed between the verbal, spoken language and the non-verbal language, called "body language." For example: in body language, a tight mouth and clenched lips express the concept of "dissatisfaction" or "withheld anger," and biting one's lips expresses concern or warning. Wing (1981), in discussing the characteristics typical of Asperger's (ASD), also notes a weak awareness and poor implementation of the non-verbal aspects of communication. She emphasizes facial expressions and gestures and the difficulty in recognizing them. Molcho (1998) and Glass (2006) include, as part of non-verbal communication, comprehending bodily signals in their entirety and perceiving what underlies voice and speech, beyond its evident content. According to Piaget (1963), our intelligence shapes the world through organization and adaptation. Merging basic sensory and movement components consists of assimilation and suitability. Thus, the link between the self and the environment is formed. A dynamic brain mechanism, responsible for merging and separation, helps to create a schema that enables structure and meaning in a person's experiences.

Adults with Asperger's (ASD) are limited in their ability to effectively apply the systems of organization and adaptation and construct the encoding and representation of their experiences. The limitations of the intrapersonal and neuro-biological dynamics are manifested in their dependency upon verbal language. This fact diminishes their sources of learning about themselves and their surroundings.

Indeed, typically, these individuals are skilled in verbal communication and in transmitting **factual information** – which may be expressed by reporting information void of any experiential shadings, and managing new information via logical processes, wherein the conclusion includes defined information. In contrast, the inability to decipher accepted social communication patterns minimizes their ability to enjoy rewarding social experiences.

The ability to read people demands being able to stop, look and listen, as a precondition for developing insights about human beings. It demands awareness and sensitivity to the signals of body language, in order to identify them in ourselves and in others in everyday life and deduce from them perceptions and significance. To better illustrate the extent of the deficiency in adults with Asperger's (ASD) of the ability to utilize the medium of non-verbal communication, let us resume a more in-depth discussion about reading people and body language.

Deriving meaning from speech, beyond its verbal content, comes from understanding facial expressions, hand gestures, voice, tone and body posture, both in ourselves and our partner in conversation. Even the pace and nuance of one's voice illuminate emotions and connotations. Glass (2006) maintains that expressing emotions is the most significant communication between human beings. The role of verbal language is to report our subjective experiences and use this channel for contact, connecting and mutual understanding.

Glass (2006) notes the importance of being attuned to verbal expressions and vocal sounds (a sigh, a cry of joy, muttering, etc.), as a means of understanding a person's emotional state (self-esteem, mischievousness, selfishness, etc.). The speaker's verbal speech pattern is also of significance and one should observe whether the speaker is slandering, cunning, vindictive, arrogant, etc., reading "between the lines." In this manner, we can also identify whether the speaker is emotionally able to find interest in his conversational partner, to pick up and understand whether he feels threatened, is mocking, thinks only in "black and white," etc. For adults with Asperger's (ASD), being able to grasp this type of information is very limited, due to above-mentioned reasons. No less important, most of them **avoid eye contact**, which is a basic precondition for picking up any kind of communication signals.

Glass (2006) specifies that people with a callous manner of speech undermine communication and contact (their tone may be narcissistic, manipulative, arrogant, ambiguous, or overstepping boundaries). She emphasizes that they are unaware of the impact of their remarks **on the other,** as they lack basic social skills. This also includes those who interrupt someone else and break his line of thought.

All this creates chaos and emotional distancing and undermines the communication process and creating contact.

Christopher (Haddon, 2003) demonstrates how the deficiencies in understanding non-verbal communication limit his capacity for adaptation. "When people tell you what to do, it's usually confusing and not logical, like for instance, when they tell me to be quiet, they don't say for how long, but when they tell me precisely what's forbidden, I like that"; "When a new teacher comes to school, I follow him with my eyes until I'm sure that he's not dangerous"; "I asked myself if it's a joke, because I don't understand jokes. When people tell jokes, they don't really mean what they say"; "I don't like reading novels, they're just lies about things that never happened." And all this, despite his normal intelligence.

Inherent in these examples are the effect of the difficulties in integrating different communication channels, the dependency upon verbal language, the complexity in evaluating the emotional state of the other, the weakness of a core coherence and informative reportage that lacks all experiential shading. These difficulties prevent Christopher from being able to adapt himself to the accepted patterns of communication.

Glass (2006) states that a person's voice intonation and nuances serve as a significant barometer for that person's sense about himself and those around him. They express despondency, support, happiness, satisfaction, tension, inner conflict, etc. They allow one to ascertain that body and speech are in harmony. For example: "I'm mad" spoken in a humorous tone will have us react with a smile. In contrast, adults with the syndrome may be confused, as they will find it difficult to decipher the contradictions inherent in this communication. Therefore, understanding vocal nuances is an important tool in interpersonal communication.

Lacking this skill, our hero Christopher experienced an encounter in a crowded train station in his own unique way: "A man came up to me and said, 'It seems you got lost', so I took out my Swiss penknife and leaned against a wall so that no one could touch me." Christopher failed to identify the support in the stranger's tone of voice, and therefore felt threatened. Glass (2006) bases voice analysis on four criteria: the height of the tone, its force, its quality (crude, shaky, pampering, etc.), and style (monotonous, sweetish, excited, etc.). She details and emphasizes that a loud voice or a soft voice both express a search for attention, that a shaky voice indicates anger or anxiety, a coarse, rough voice usually indicates hard, unloving people, and a sexy voice is linked to being insincere and manipulative. And these are just a few of the examples. Glass further states that reading body language or facial expressions may be a more successful barometer than the words spoken, as a person's face is the bulletin board of his inner soul.

Christopher relates that when his Dad hit the steering-wheel with his fist, I knew he was angry, because he was also yelling. It isn't hard to imagine the father's facial expression that preceded this drama. But to Christopher it related very little. Parents of children with the syndrome testify that their message doesn't sink in until they raise their voice to a strong enough pitch that creates drama.

According to Molcho (1998), body language plays a significant role in interpersonal communication. It serves as a stimulus for the person and facilitates expressing his reactions accordingly. Therefore, it is important that we be aware that what our body broadcasts has an impact on others.

This chapter is about the importance of messages that are transmitted via non-verbal communication, which is a complex process of looks, movements and various types of gestures. The meaning of the communication message is usually understood through an integration of all that is happening at a given moment of interpersonal interaction.

People with Asperger's (ASD) have a hard time paying attention, absorbing, understanding, interpreting and integrating the codes, gestures, emotions and other signals, and therefore **the problem is complex and challenging.** Nevertheless, the non-verbal language repertoire can be improved and even expanded by applying communication exercises.

Adults with Asperger's (ASD) communicate well, using verbal language. However, naturally, interpersonal communication is constructed from a variety of paths. Duck (1986), in his book *Human Relationships*, calls them the hidden languages of social behavior. He asserts that these languages render interpersonal verbal communication to be more efficient and are therefore vital in every relationship. Molcho (1998) reinforces this viewpoint in saying that body language opens direct paths to other people. In fact, our picture of reality is created via collecting and sorting different impressions.

Duck (1986) claims that non-verbal communication plays the role of regulating and refining social behavior. Using this language helps transmit messages, beyond the content and meaning of the words.

Glass asserts that a person is a complete story that can be read by his voice, manner of speech, face, movements and bodily posture. Together, they provide clues to the inner reality of ourselves and others.

A story related in a parents' support group illustrates how the "blindness" in reading people undermines the ability to develop empathy: The youngest daughter of the family dreamed of becoming a pianist and began studying piano at a relatively young age. Her face shone whenever she spoke of this to others and when she practiced on the piano. Her older brother decided that she must be told "the truth," so that she doesn't live in an illusion. He told her that he didn't think she played that well and that she would never become a pianist. The young girl cried and mourned her dream, and never played again.

Her brother saw only the facts, without reading her inner reality. This pattern repeated itself in his places of employment and he was forced to change jobs frequently as a result.

This story and others like it illustrate the expression: "Walking with eyes closed along the highway of life," which typifies the communication experiences of adults with Asperger's (ASD).

Glass (2006), a psychologist specializing in this field, emphasizes and sharpens what it is that is demanded of each one of us in order to successfully "ford the river" of interpersonal communication. It comprises the barriers and obstacles that people with Asperger's (ASD) are confronted with. In her book, she details dozens of signals and stimuli that we must pay attention to and must absorb and interpret as we communicate with others. As she explains, they have to be felt and the significance of each one must be read as well. The multi-linked chain of failures experienced by adults with Asperger's (ASD) begins with the neuro-biological deficiency and the core symptoms. It begins with the difficulty in creating eye contact, in dealing with multiple stimuli and integrating them into a meaningful experience.

Correspondingly, it is hard for them to identify their own emotions, as well as that of others, and express them. This is a major factor, highly important in assuring the flow of communication. The emotional effort that an adult with the syndrome must invest in an interpersonal and social encounter, and his subsequent frustration, are much greater than anything neurotypical people could possibly imagine.

Meyer (2001) is a project director, researcher and writer of the Asperger's (ASD), ever since he himself was diagnosed with the syndrome at a late age. He testifies from his own experience that people with the syndrome find it hard to do multitasking, which also impacts on their coping with interpersonal communication. Eating with others, Meyer writes, is a challenge with many obstacles. Eating in itself is a multi-sensory task, and eating socially requires carrying out complex social ceremonies. Therefore, people with Asperger's (ASD) try to eat alone, even in situations where eating alone is not the norm. Meyer (2001) explains: "We find it hard to uncover the right clues while we are searching for the mandatory rules and customs." Added to this is the inability to observe an event from its different facets and a decreased ability for "playing along" or thought association. Herein also lies the barrier to understanding humor, metaphors, joking around, pranks and variations of the language. Frith (1991) notes that these failures grow out of a reduced ability to think coherently. This concept relates to the ability to carry out systematic integration between different types of information, identify their relationship to the matter at hand and create clarity, understanding and meaningfulness. All these impact upon the everyday life of adults with Asperger's (ASD). Clinging to a familiar meaning bars the ability to relate to the event or experience as it actually unfolds at any given time and place, and respond in a relevant manner. This phenomenon has been conceptualized as a pragmatic difficulty. For example, a student who was studying engineering in college stood out as someone with inflexible integrity, which was to his detriment. To his understanding, the lecturer tended to favor two of the students in class. To him this seemed unjust, so he stood up in class and protested to the lecturer bluntly in front of all the students. The lecturer, who was angry and insulted, called him to the college director's office for a talk and he was warned that if such behavior were repeated, he would be expelled from the college.

This student, apparently, had a basic misunderstanding of the system in which he was studying. It was reflected in his misguided perception of authoritarian relationships. Additionally, he lacked the strategic skills in the social system, with which he could have planned a request for a personal meeting with the lecturer, instead of embarrassing him in front of his students. His disability to understand signals that are beyond the spoken word and integrate all the signs was his downfall and prevented him from correctly estimating the social system he was part of and the consequences of his actions.

A further example: a young man in his late twenties traveled abroad with his parents on frequent occasions. Even though the airport was clearly a familiar place, the security check caused him anxiety each time anew, as he believed he was under suspicion. This intelligent adult found it hard to understand the context of the situation and the systemic principles that set it in motion, and so he developed futile anxiety and a temporary sense of persecution regarding all that transpired at the airport. Therefore, It is not hard to assume that his reactions and behavior were also inappropriate and did not meet the accepted social norms.

Serious attention must be given to the extensive suffering caused to adults with Asperger's (ASD) by the multi-limbed "octopus" of difficulties in complex and multiple-channeled communication, which neurotypical people cope with successfully for the most part. If we step into the shoes of these adults with the syndrome, we will be able to feel, to some extent, how they are "groping in the dark," so long as they are required to communicate, connect with and cooperate with other people. Additionally, we will be able to increase our empathy for their helplessness, the outcome of their relative lack of skills in understanding what is transpiring simultaneously in multiple dimensions. This is of great importance, because uncertainty is a catalyst for anxiety, and ongoing anxiety promotes increased depression.

Even though the difficulties in communication for people with Asperger's (ASD) are anchored in their neuro-biological deficiency, a communication bridge can be built, and teaching the general norms of interpersonal communication, via understanding, support, tolerance and encouragement, will upgrade their quality of life.

CHAPTER 3

SOCIAL AND INTERPERSONAL DIFFICULTIES – CAUSES, PROCESSES, OUTCOMES AND IMPLICATIONS

INTRODUCTION

Tantam, (in Klin et al, 2000) reports that a significant percentage of those referred to his clinic had been previously diagnosed with various and strange psychiatric diagnoses for which they received superfluous medication. This painful experience is common among people with Asperger's (ASD) and their families, for when they were growing up, the syndrome had not yet been defined.

A comprehensive review of the literature relating to Asperger's (ASD) shows that there is agreement between the experts that the basic deficiency in this field is neuro-biological in origin. Today, research carried out on the brain functions of people with the syndrome provides documentation that this is a congenital developmental syndrome with a genetic component. Attwood notes [2007] that there are families who have multiple relatives with Asperger's (ASD), as well as families in which the syndrome appears to have skipped a generation.

The aim of the discussion in this chapter is to focus on and sort the known characteristics of the syndrome and examine the reciprocal effect of the symptoms and their repercussion on everyday life.

The neuro-biological deficiency is at the core of the syndrome and it is there for life. It is also why adults with the syndrome suffer from functional disorders and grow up feeling they are different and socially challenged. They absorb repeated blows, such as rejection, mockery, loneliness and failure. Secondary manifestations also kick in, triggered by the effort to survive and avoid pain. Attwood notes that each person is an individual with a unique cluster of symptoms of one kind or another, and that each person is on another point along the spectrum. However, social deficiency is something that all those diagnosed with Asperger's (ASD) share in common.

SOCIAL DEFICIENCY – ITS SOURCES AND OUTCOMES

Social and interpersonal deficiency is a complex deficiency with multiple implications and outcomes. It typifies all adults with Asperger's (ASD) and is unique to this syndrome.

Goleman (2007) in his book, *Social Intelligence*, describes the social mind as a system containing all the neurological mechanisms that modify our communication, thoughts and feelings toward others, and set in motion our relationships with others. Social intelligence, in his view, is the ability of one person to look beyond individual perception, in order to understand what is taking place in the interaction between people. This skill is deficient in people with Asperger's (ASD), as the neurological system in their "social mind" functions differently.

Goleman builds his theory upon the assumption that the mutuality in interpersonal communication is built along two channels: The higher channel – in which calculated understanding of what is happening in reality takes place, and the lower channel – in which the immediate intuitive response to the other takes place. The higher channel helps us decipher what took place, following the experience and the intuitive response, and consolidates their significance. Thus, our social life is navigated by the mutuality between these two channels, which together create social awareness and skills. He points out that damage to the emotional sphere disturbs the capability for synchronization, empathy, social awareness and communication skills.

Convincing testimony came from a young man who, following two years of psychological treatment, informed his therapist that he has Asperger's (ASD). When asked, "How is that?," he told her that he happened to come across an article on the internet, and there he learned that people with the syndrome are unable to identify or define what they feel. He claimed that for a long time he has been aware of having feelings without understanding what they are. Further testing confirmed the diagnosis. Which is to say: If someone with the syndrome is unable to identify his own emotions, how could he possibly understand what another person is feeling? The lack of understanding of the feelings and thoughts of others precludes any emotional mutuality and encumbers social and communication reciprocity. Therefore, when encountering a conversation between two or more people, those with the syndrome find it hard to take part in the dialogue, which involves the spontaneous sharing of experiences. The behavior that typifies them is to state their presence via a one-sided "lecture" about their special field of interest, inundating the listeners with details, totally unaware to what extent – if at all – they are interested, paying attention, are tired or are in a rush to leave. At a social event, I met a middle-aged man who illustrated this most concretely – he talked endlessly about his favorite topic and clearly was enjoying himself. When someone finally managed to divert the conversation to another topic, his face fell, he withdrew into himself and remained silent.

Tantam, (in Frith 1991), asserts that Asperger's (ASD) must be assumed as a possible diagnosis for anyone who encounters difficulties in his communication, sociality and mutuality, and whose developmental history points to phenomena in this area from early childhood. This syndrome is a malfunction of the reflexes of observing and paying attention to social cues from infancy.

One of the mothers in a parents' support group related how she had suspected that her baby girl had hearing problems, because she didn't respond to the human voice. However, hearing tests negated that. When she was two years old, the little girl still would not turn her head when her name was called. She grew up with difficulties in social adaptation and was later diagnosed with Asperger's (ASD).

MALFUNCTIONS IN EMPATHY AS A CRITICAL BARRIER

The definition of 'empathy' in the *Dictionary of Psychology* (Reber, A. S.) is the absorption of the feelings and perspective of another, as well as the understanding that enables a person to comprehend what his fellow man is going through. All this takes place through a process in which viewpoints and feelings are transmitted from one person to another, even without verbal communication. The neurological malfunctioning of people with Asperger's (ASD) may impede the ability to comprehend the emotional echoing of the other, thus preventing empathic communication from developing. An empathic experience begins to form when emotional resonance is felt, creating an infrastructure for dialogue and connection. The adult with ASD syndrome finds it hard to express understanding, resulting from his difficulty to identify and define his own feelings and those of another person. Empathy creates a bond ("chemistry") between the dialogue participants and enables each participant to experience emotional sharing between himself and the other.

In the empathic experience, one side has understanding vis-à-vis the feelings, thoughts, intentions, goals and also pain of the other, without identifying with him nor feeling the same as he. Empathy is an important element in interpersonal connections and social belonging (Baron-Cohen, et all, 1995).

The lack of empathic sensitivity constitutes an obstacle toward understanding social codes, from several aspects: When interacting, a person diagnosed with Asperger's (ASD) finds it difficult to understand the context, to decode what is happening, to recognize its significance and to respond accordingly. For those with the syndrome, a social experience is fraught with uncertainty, anxieties and frustrations. From the amassed sediments of previous failures in social situations, a variety of feelings arise, a sense of not belonging, of estrangement. A person with ASD syndrome seeks protection from failure and pain by avoiding involvement with people and develops a tendency toward seclusion.

Robison (2007) admits that his sensitivity to what others are doing is limited to such a degree that "if a woman tried to flirt with me, I didn't notice." He relates how many of his relationships fell apart due to his unconventional style of communication, and the fact that he was alone because of his disability was one of the most bitter disappointments in his young life.

This situation accompanied him up to adulthood, even after he became aware of Asperger's (ASD). He was clever, gentle and funny and looked "pretty normal" but, as he relates, his behavior was apparently different. He testifies that his behavior knew no bounds, that he would ask direct and blunt questions which caused others to feel insulted. He understood that his analytic way of thinking was perceived by others as a lack of intuition and feelings (i.e., empathy) and this drove people away. Being a creative genius, he sums up, did not help in making friends and did not make him happy.

THE SEMANTIC-PRAGMATIC DIMENSION

Webster (1989) defines semantics: "The meaning or relation-ship of meanings of a sign or set of signs, especially its connota-tive meaning." The difficulties for adults with Asperger's (ASD) in the semantic dimension of language add a significant hardship to their interpersonal and social communication. They have no difficulty in understanding the meaning of words, sentences and narratives, as abstract as they may be, as long as they need only understand at the syntax level alone.

Verbal communication via clear, direct language constitutes an efficient channel for them, as long as things are spoken in a direct manner, meaning, "literally." In contrast, they find it hard to decipher allegories and sayings, slang expressions, sophisticat-ed humor and metaphors, even within everyday communication.

One of the mothers in a parents' support group related how she had asked her son, who has Asperger's (ASD), to "hop" over to the kitchen and fetch her a towel. Her adolescent son did so immediately: he reached the kitchen and returned to her...the entire time hopping on his two feet, instead of just walking. This **intelligent** adolescent had a semantic handicap, which led him to understand what was said to him at the "literal" level and was unable to perceive the symbolic meaning of the words.

A hyperactive adolescent, who attended a therapy center I directed years ago, climbed up a high roof and didn't know how to climb down. I instructed him to sit down and then jump so that he lands on his butt. This young lad took off his pants and jumped… on his butt. He too was unable to understand beyond the words' concrete meaning.

Difficulty with pragmatic thinking and language is yet another dimension that undermines their communication with the neurotypical social world. It is generally thought that their high cognitive skills enable them to comprehend, understand and use "formal" syntaxes of language at a high level. Nonetheless, they suffer from mistakes in communication. According to Reber, (1985) pragmatism is "a special reference to the **causes, the antecedent conditions** and the practical **consequences**." Webster indicates that in pragmatic language, emphasis is put on "the function of the various forms of expressions, and not just on the expression's forms in themselves. That is, upon the **use** and the **consequences** of the verbal signs and other forms of expression." In the everyday practical life of adults with Asperger's (ASD), the semantic dimension and the pragmatic dimension are intertwined.

The deficiencies in this area decrease or block the ability to observe what is happening from different perspectives and the ability for intellectual play with the contextual material (allegories, imagery, symbols and metaphors). Additionally, there is diminished ability to decipher the social map, exploit the data it provides within a changing environment and apply it with practical effectiveness.

One mother told her daughter, a girl with Asperger's (ASD), "Get a grip on yourself," and in response, the daughter hugged herself. A young man with Asperger's (ASD) was asked to go and check why the baby in the next room was screaming, and to pick her up if she had fallen. He soon returned, and the baby was still screaming. When asked why he hadn't picked her up, he answered: "Because she didn't fall." It turned out that the baby was screaming because her hand had gotten caught in a drawer.

The semantic-pragmatic dimension has ramifications that impact upon the entire spectrum of the rules of social behavior: greeting someone, reporting, requesting instead of demanding, etc. It also includes the difficulty in adjusting the language to one's conversational partner or to the situation at hand: a different form of speech with an infant as opposed to conversing with an adult, or clarifying the topic under discussion for someone who is unfamiliar with it, etc. The attending problems are linked to a limited ability to conduct oneself according to accepted rules of conversation: Waiting for one's turn to speak, staying on the subject at hand, maintaining eye contact, answering questions, focusing at one and the same time on the spoken words and body language, how and when to enter a discussion, or change the subject, etc.

Breaking these rules is considered strange and incomprehensible behavior in the social environment. It is further perceived as pretended innocence, annoyance or stupidity and may give rise to anger, judgmental criticism or rejection. Since the adult with Asperger's (ASD) does not understand where he went wrong and why others are angry at him, he is left without any means of coping and remains hurt and anxious.

A young couple, both with Asperger's (ASD), went to the cinema. As they were waiting in line to buy tickets, a young woman in front of them suddenly felt ill, fell down and fainted. When one of the standers-by bent over her to help her, the young lady from this couple reacted hysterically and screamed: "Help! Rape!"

The pragmatic malfunction constitutes a stumbling block for

people with the syndrome in adjusting to independent living within society, sometimes to the point where they become unintentionally involved in small encounters with the law. This is because the semantic-pragmatic barrier undermines their ability to foresee the results of their actions and the harm their behavior may cause.

MUTUALITY – AN EXISTENTIAL ISSUE IN INTERPERSONAL AND SOCIAL RELATIONSHIPS.

Mutuality is expressed via commitment and involvement in activities, opinions, feelings, ideas and support between two or more people. Mutuality is of especial importance when one side balances out the other, both emotionally and practically, via a process of give-and-take. The fact that involvement between adult persons is based on the principle of give-and-take is common knowledge. The nature of the relationship is what determines the conditions and the essence of implementing this principle, and requires the cooperation and agreement of all the sides involved. The connection between people, whatever it be, may not be sustained over a long period of time if the principle of give-and-take does not withstand the test of mutuality.

People with Asperger's (ASD) are highly capable of verbal expression, but a closer look will reveal that they have barriers in communication and in connecting with others, which undermine their ability to promote cooperation and mutuality.

In fact, their difficulty in understanding and applying mutual relationships is **the result** of the mix of various symptoms of the syndrome, which dictate their blatant tendency toward individualism and seclusion. This mix includes neuro-biological, neuro-psychological and emotional manifestations and a variety of survival mechanisms.

Mutuality cannot exist without social awareness, it is the range between the immediate and intuitive perception of what a person has experienced and understanding his intentions, feelings and thoughts, to the deciphering of more complex social situations. Stanford (2006) asserts that this is linked to a defense mechanism. She disagrees with those who hold that if enjoyment is not shared – there is no enjoyment, and claims that the difference in people with ASD syndrome lies in their not getting any enjoyment from spontaneous sharing in itself.

Based on my understanding of the origins of Asperger's (ASD), the obstacle to inclusion and spontaneity derives, in part at least, from the neurological malfunction. Indeed, a lack of communicative spontaneity is a prominent trait among people on the autistic spectrum. According to Stanford's understanding (2006), emotional mutuality is the give-and-take of the emotional world. Emotional mutuality is the main support that insures a stable, ongoing relationship.

Even when an adult with Asperger's (ASD) has been able to internalize over the years the basic significance of social interaction, there still may appear misunderstandings regarding the sophisticated nature of giving and taking in the reciprocal relations between adults.

Robison (2007), in his autobiography, shares with us that at times, he can can relate to a machine better than to people. Machines can be controlled regardless of their size and they are predictable. He says that he has problems reading people and that he cannot **look at** people and know if they like him are angry, or are just waiting for him to speak.

This description contains only a small number of the obstacles that people with the syndrome encounter. In their efforts to connect and communicate with others, it is important to emphasize here once again their difficulty in deciphering social codes, in learning rules of behavior, in knowing how to read the social map, etc. As he testifies: "It was hard for me to live with all the people in one house, I didn't know what to say or what to do, and I felt lost."

Mutuality in general, and emotional mutuality specifically, cannot develop without a basis of empathic abilities of all those involved, wherein each of the persons can sense in one way or another the emotional state of the other or others.

Mutuality is also important for a utilitarian relationship, which is a connection with others in order to achieve a practical, implemental or material goal. Mutuality is needed in relationships in order to set in motion everyday life. All of us are involved in utilitarian relationships. However, where one of the partners has Asperger's (ASD), mutuality is especially significant in order to maintain that relationship.

CHAPTER 4

ADULT LIFE ACCORDING TO ASPERGER'S (ASD)

There are a number of personality traits that are characteristic of people with ASD syndrome. Traits such as frankness and morality reflect the personality of a person with integrity. These traits, together with good cognitive skills, can contribute to improving the quality of life of an adult who must cope with the challenges.

However, for adults with Asperger's (ASD) this is a mixed blessing, and it is not self-evident. They are unaware of the principles upon which social norms are based, therefore they don't tend to behave according to those conventions and find it hard to apply them from one situation to another and include them in new situations.

Their difficulty with the neurotypical rules of behavior is also linked to understanding the intentions and goals of the conversational partner. I recall the story of a young, lonely man who one day knocked on the office door of a senior manager's office where he worked. She was married and the mother of children, but he knocked on her door to confess his love to her. Despite the fact that he was an efficient and industrious worker, he was fired the following day. His behavior crossed the boundaries of the system's ability to contain and digest it. Sometime later, the young man was diagnosed as fitting the definition of a person with Asperger's (ASD).

Interpersonal and social malfunctioning is at times revealed at its greatest impact when one needs to cope with the demands of adulthood, according to Szatmari (in Klin et al., 2006). After completing their education, some adults with Asperger's (ASD) continue to reside in their parents' home, unemployed. Others may find themselves residing in a halfway house suited to their needs, if their community provides it. Their quality of life is influenced by their perception of their condition, and the extent to which they aspire to develop social contact and feel they have successfully accomplished it.

The interpersonal behavior of adults with Asperger's (ASD) is often interpreted by the surrounding environment as abnormal and strange. Various reactions toward them may be exclusion, mockery and name-calling, and some of these adults encounter such badgering in their workplaces as well. They tend to fail in integrating socially into the framework, and lack the skills that could serve them effectively in initiating a process to correct the situation. Appropriately, these skills should be imbued as soon as the young adults leave the educational frameworks.

One of my neighbors told me that her adult son was diagnosed with Asperger's (ASD), and since then a new dialogue has developed between them and they have renewed the connection between them. This was a most significant step for them, as prior to that, the son was often angry, but since the diagnosis, his mother has been helping him and he has made progress in his ability to adjust to social frameworks.

Our clinical experience points to the need for professional help after leaving institutional frameworks, as the adult with the syndrome tends to withdraw into a comfortable bubble, free of the incomprehensible "noises" outside in the social world. This withdrawal helps protect them from failures and the accompanying pain. Inside this safe "bubble" they develop a narrow area of interest, in which they become engrossed and at which they become expert. This enables some of them to be employed in a variety of technical fields, such as computers, developing and repairing apparatus and devices, but also in the fields of philosophy, science, music, etc. Glen Gould, the renowned pianist, retired from public appearances at the height of his career. He withdrew to his home in a, preferring a life of seclusion and complete addiction to piano playing. This lifestyle does not help people with the syndrome to cope with their problems and to seek help in finding ways to adjust to the world in order to achieve a fuller adult life. Based on data collected to date, it can be said that the developmental profile of the adult with Asperger's (ASD) is different from that of neurotypical adults. Though most of them very much desire to have a social life and intimacy, only very few succeed in connecting and becoming part of a social network, or find a permanent relationship with another.

They don't have a consolidated emotional and social awareness, and their logical thinking skills – which in themselves are very good – contribute little to their interpersonal functioning. Observing their social behavior further clarifies this gap.

Asperger's (ASD) is indeed an elusive syndrome. We are dealing here with a population of adults who are generally well educated. Many of them successfully graduated from high schools and colleges within the normal stream of education, yet did not succeed in fitting in socially. However, they are not sentenced to a life of isolation and loneliness. Today, accumulated experience indicates that they are capable of improving their social adaptation even in adulthood.

Additionally, the accumulative experience of clinicians indicates that these adults can be taught the norms required in order to cope for survival socially and professionally, and that training toward interpersonal skills and developing social proficiencies is beneficial to adults with the syndrome. Those with weakened empathy as well can learn to strengthen their ability to identify and use their own feelings, as well as those of others, and utilize them in order to connect and form human relationships.

There is great importance, therefore, in the new development among professionals involved in the treatment and rehabilitation of the population diagnosed with Asperger's (ASD), to remain updated in understanding the complex makeup of the fabric of life of adults with ASD syndrome.

CHAPTER 5

POTENTIAL CAUSES OF DIFFICULTIES IN ADAPTATION FOR ADULTS WITH ASPERGER'S (ASD)

In discussing the causes that impact on the adults' adaptation difficulties, the issues involved include a range of phenomena. In therapeutic work, we discover that each individual has his own unique profile, which includes potential abilities, personality structure and environmental influences. Stanford (2006) holds that in order to help adults with Asperger's (ASD) to survive as well as succeed, they must receive the support of others. This includes family and friends, treatment and rehabilitation frameworks.

In order for them to cope with a variety of hardships, support networks are needed that can provide guidance and encouragement within facilitating frameworks. They need a comfort zone in which they are accepted with respect and understanding. Under conditions in which the supportive elements recognize and confirm individual capabilities, one's self-confidence can be boosted to facilitate motivation and ability in coping with the challenges. These are prerequisites for growth and empowerment that will enable the adult with ASD syndrome to seek and find the way to achieve a balance between his need to protect himself and his desire for change.

In order to help adults with Asperger's (ASD) rehabilitate successfully, it is of utmost importance that therapists, rehabilitation professionals, educators, **employers,** friends, and those within family circles attain an empathic understanding of the syndrome. Concurrently, they should approach each such adult as having a unique cluster of symptoms, and identify those areas that demand special efforts in order to understand his **individual** adaptation difficulties. It is essential to keep in mind that the syndrome is the result of congenital developmental factors.

I recently heard of a man with ASD syndrome who knew by heart the names of most of the soccer players on the teams from Israel and throughout the world. However, he had no interest in the game of soccer itself and had no idea of what really takes place on the field. His attempts to join conversations about soccer were unsuccessful. In his book, Meyers (2001) specifies unusual behaviorisms that are characterized by reduction and obsessiveness: Preferring a limited selection of clothing items; feeling uncomfortable in formal clothes; preferences or strong aversions to specific foods, along with a strict adherence to inflexible and unaccepted eating habits (such as choosing to eat alone with no others present). A tolerant approach can help ease a feeling of strangeness and provide the freedom to be oneself. Perhaps it is through the experience of an accepting environment that the adult with ASD syndrome will be able to open to change.

MOTORIC CLUMSINESS AND SENSORY SENSITIVITY

Klin et al (2001) present research indicating that part of the autistic population displays clumsiness. Their physical awkwardness is mostly expressed via body movements. Adults with Asperger's (ASD) usually possess a good level of spatial vision, yet their hand-eye coordination is characteristically somewhat problematic.

I personally experienced this reality when a young man with the syndrome came to meet with me. He quickly dropped his heavy frame into the armchair, which "groaned" and squeaked under his weight. In order to ease his embarrassment, I led the discussion to what had just happened. He soon revealed that he is similarly embarrassed by the fact that when he pours milk into his coffee, the coffee spills over. When that happens, other family members get angry with him, believing it is because of carelessness and disdain, even though they now know that he is diagnosed with Asperger's (ASD). They don't understand that he tries to prevent this from happening but doesn't succeed.

Uncommon sensory experiences characterize many adults with Asperger's (ASD). They may be sensitive or unusually insensitive to smell, noise, temperature, touch, light, pain, taste and other sensory stimuli, and some may have sleeping disorders. Thus, if a person with the syndrome attends a family celebration or other social gathering that is filled with blinding lights, loud music and everyone talking to one another, he will find it hard to adjust.

When the stimuli are overwhelming, people with the syndrome will revert to self-stimulatory behavior (stims) to increase their sense of self-control and reduce tension and anxiety. Examples of this could be waving their hands about without any communicative aim, nail-biting, raising one's voice, their thoughts wandering (they seem to be daydreaming) and even total detachment or walking to and fro while talking to oneself. These and other such behaviorisms are often observed in people with ASD syndrome. Additionally, there may be loss of control following a sensory or multitasking overload.

They become stressed out from interruptions to whatever they are doing, or from contradictory and confusing demands. These can lead to extreme reactions of anger in order to free themselves of the confusion and control the situation. The following incident illustrates this well: In a certain high school one of the youngsters, who was diagnosed with Asperger's (ASD), was unable to contain and digest everything that was happening in school. When the stimuli surrounding him became overwhelming, he would leave class and stand in the corridor and scream as loudly as he could. When asked why he did this, he said: "If I don't scream, how will anyone know that I'm suffering?"

This illustrates how deep and complex the syndrome is. This youngster, who was intelligent and able to deal with the high school studies, as far as what was required at the academic level of the learned materials, was unable to contain the sensory stimuli and the multitasking demands placed upon him. He furthermore felt frustrated as he did not meet his expectations from himself in regard to his social integration. He was incapable of expressing his emotional distress in an accepted manner. Due to the difficulty in identifying, expressing and communicating his feelings, the only path left for him was to scream out his distress.

Prince-Hughes (2006) describes in her book, with captivating simplicity and directness, her own sensory experiences and how she coped with them. She relates that she had a strong reaction to noises and lights. She didn't like to be held, and drew back if someone tried to hug her. She also didn't like the touch of the carpet or bare floor. She was addicted to odors and touching sensations, she had a craving for salt, would suck on burned matches and loved the smell of the car. The clink of a teaspoon or sound of a clock excited her, yet other sounds were painful. Prince-Hughs loved repetitiveness and symmetry, order and ceremony; she insisted on always taking the same route and hated any change, because "it was like murder." She wore leather clothes because their weight calmed her and wore sunglasses even at night in order to decrease stimuli. She relates how, as a result of the syndrome, she felt as if she were drowning in an ocean that is unpredictable, with no landmarks or shores. The effort to introduce order into the chaos in any possible way constitutes a defense mechanism for self-preservation.

The growing body of proof of the inability to fit in and be "normal," the memories and pain – all these are compensated for via compulsive behavior and rigidity. In *The Curious Incident of the Dog in the Night-Time* (Haddon, 2003), there is a highly informative description by Christopher, the story's hero, of coping with sensory malfunctions that lead to overload. He relates how, when people were too close to him and the noise was strong inside his head, he found it difficult to think, as if someone were screaming inside his head. In order to survive, he would walk along the edge of the road, cover his ears and groan. Further on he relates that when he finds himself in a new place where there are a lot of people, he covers his ears to keep out the noise and think. He then feels as if he has shut down the computer and then reboots it, in order to remember "what I am doing and where I'm supposed to go."

OPPORTUNITIES VIS-À-VIS BARRIERS: ABILITIES VIS-À-VIS DIFFICULTIES

Stanford (2001) raises the conjecture that a lack of social experience leads to the onset of a low self-image and an unconsolidated identity. Thus, for people with Asperger's (ASD), being able to engage in social and interpersonal reciprocal relationships is no minor matter: From early childhood they have experienced negative labeling from their environment, such as "lone wolf," "genius," "asocial," "rigid," "nerd," etc. This name-calling is repeated so long as the social situation they are trying to connect to is not receptive of them. Thus they reach adulthood, with their self so deeply scarred that both body and mind do not forget. Their self-image and social confidence remain impaired.

Prince-Hughes (2006), in her autobiographical book, *Songs of the Gorilla Nation*, relates how she was diagnosed at the age of 36 and the fact that she had survived seemed miraculous to her. She asserts that the functioning adults with ASD syndrome don't know "what's wrong" with them and use their intelligence in order to appear to be "like everyone else." Society expects from a person with Asperger's (ASD) to understand and conduct himself without guidance. Prince-Hughes describes the outcome from her own personal experience: "I was embarrassed by not knowing what to do and the presence of another person made me anxious. In such a case, I would either leave or become insolent." Robison (2007), in his autobiographical book, relates that during his first few years of life, his parents took him to a dozen different mental health professionals, and "instead of looking at me through sympathetic lenses, the professionals said I was lazy, ill-tempered and rebellious." The social awareness of a neurotypical person provides him with the skills required to create for himself supportive networks in his human environment. In contrast, people with Asperger's (ASD) absorb extensive mockery and rejection from society throughout their life and as a result they develop fears and a tendency toward avoidance. They are, therefore, in need of a supportive network as a tool to help them repair their confusion and relieve their worries. Prince-Hughes noticed that adults with the syndrome long to have others confirm their experiences and relate to them. She relates how her partner would interpret for her human behavior and its rules, and explain to her where she went wrong, when she committed a social mistake. Slowly she began to understand the behavior codes. It is generally accepted that seeking support is a basic human need. However, those diagnosed with ASD syndrome need to be connected to and supported by people who are familiar with and understand the syndrome.

Attwood, in the introduction to Meyer's book (2001), asserts that adults with Asperger's (ASD) require guidance throughout their employment years, guidance that will focus on those areas that need reinforcement and maintenance. Meyer claims that adults with the syndrome who internalize it as a neurological anomaly are more capable of appreciating the importance of their abilities and think of themselves as whole people who can contribute to society.

These adults are intelligent, with unique talents and skills, and with special fields of interest in which they tend to invest a lot and become very knowledgeable. These talents can potentially be translated into a prospering career. However, as of now, only some of these adults remain in their jobs and many of them do not fulfill their potential.

In this regard, the following are the profiles of two adults with ASD syndrome, which reflect their abilities and the difficulties blocking their potential opportunities. The first profile is that of a young man in his twenties: He studied history and political science at the university and has acquired extensive knowledge in these fields, which also stimulate his interest and curiosity. He is skilled in verbal expression and is good at process analyses. However, he is unable to apply these skills in professional employment, due to attention deficit and a tendency to disengage, difficulty in practical organization and clumsiness.

The second profile is of a man in his late thirties: He has academic degrees in engineering and a wide knowledge in technical fields. Practically, as well, his technical skills are highly developed and he is outstanding at assembling, building and repairing machines and apparatus of all kinds. Additionally, he has a superb memory for details, high curiosity in the fields that interest him and a tendency toward inquisitiveness. Perseverance and determination, loyalty, integrity, honesty and reliability are his outstanding qualities. However, people cause him great distress, he does not make eye contact; when he talks to someone, he doesn't notice that the other person isn't listening; he finds it hard to participate in small talk; eats only specific foods, and always wears the same type of clothing. These manifestations have accompanied him since early childhood.

Most adults with Asperger's (ASD) do not establish families due to the hardships in connecting to a partner. Some accounts indicate that among those who are married, there is a high divorce rate. Though there are couples who remain together and establish a proper family, it is noteworthy – as also seen when reading Stanford's book (2006) (Stanford's partner is a man with Asperger's (ASD)) – that usually the partner is someone who is supportive, holding, flexible and tolerant, who enables his or her partner "to be themselves," as he or she were meant to be.

According to Stanford, due to the difficulty in establishing and maintaining a relationship as a couple, on the one hand, and integrating into an employment network, on the other hand, a significant portion of the adults with Asperger's (ASD) are prevented from progressing and developing in the course of their lives and realizing their hidden potential.

CHAPTER 6

ABOUT ASPERGER'S (ASD) AND EMOTIONS

Asperger's (ASD) is an elusive syndrome. The cognitive abilities of people with the syndrome builds expectations in relation to their emotional and social functioning. As a result, every failure or shortcoming in their social and interpersonal skills can be misleading and even confusing to those around them. In response, an adult with ASD lives with the feeling that he is a disappointment to the most significant people in his life, as well as to himself. Frequently, he does not understand where he went wrong and what are the causes **and consequences** of his behavior. Lacking diagnosis and treatment, the hardships that these adults endure become highly arduous.

Klin (Klin et al., 2000) specifies the neurological processes involved. The mechanism in the brain that connects the emotional dimension to an experienced event is, most likely, responsible for the interpretation of human facial expressions and creates the neurological synchronization with an emotional experience. When this neurological mechanism does not function properly, the person with ASD has a difficult time observing and identifying emotions that are expressed both facially and bodily. Thus, from early childhood, he is denied the opportunities to learn from personal experience how to develop interpersonal ties.

Baron-Cohen (Baron-Cohen et al, 1997) submitted a model that claims that we read another person's mind all the time, automatically, mostly unconsciously. Reading one's mind is the natural way to understand, interpret and also respond with the appropriate social behavior. Neurotypical adults attribute to others emotional states, such as thoughts, feelings, passions and intentions. Baron-Cohen and his colleagues state that human beings developed neuro-cognitive mechanisms that facilitate reading one's mind, to link rational thinking to actions and interpret looks as significant gestures. In this regard, they developed the concept TOM (Theory of mind), which defines our ability to create a theory of what is taking place in the mind of another person. For adults with Asperger's (ASD), the early failures to transfer social and emotional knowledge to mental and motoric centers, along with wrong responses to social stimuli, hinder their ability to communicate emotional and social information. It is these early failures that may give rise to a chain of events in which erroneous social reference exists.

The world of emotions is a rich totality of basic and universal emotions, consisting of clusters of feelings and emotional shadings that are personal and subjective. For adults with ASD, the disruption in those channels that connect an experienced emotion to the mental and motoric centers, causes them to be frequently perceived as odd. Testimonials to this effect, from people with Asperger's (ASD), relate how they always knew they were feeling things, but were unable to define what they were feeling. One person expressed an additional insight: "If I don't understand what I'm feeling, how can I understand what another person is feeling?"

Research confirms the fact that the neurological "short circuit" in the emotion's path, moving from internally to externally, is to be found in the channels of reception, transference and the expression of the emotion. Based on that, it might be assumed that the emotions of a person with ASD are trapped in the depths of his soul, "existent but invisible to the observer," that is, they exist but remain non-communicative. Indeed, a deceptive syndrome.

Attwood claims that when a person with Asperger's (ASD) does not have an empathic language of communication, it is wrong to assume that he is indifferent to his surroundings. It is more precise to say that he has difficulty in **deciphering** the emotions of another, as well as **expressing** his own feelings.

Parents relate how they have to be dramatic in their body language, their tone of speech and their facial expressions in order to help their child with ASD identify what it is they want or mean, and react accordingly. One mother of an adolescent boy complained that though it is possible to dramatize for him anger and frustration, communicating nuances is very difficult.

Attwood found that adults with Asperger's (ASD) are able to identify basic emotions, but have difficulty in expressing complex emotions (embarrassment, pride, etc.). Their emotional world can be compared to a field without any marked paths in it, therefore it is hard to find a path that leads to emotional and social communication and connection. Whereas the emotional experiences do exist, they remain at an impasse and cause emotional distress. The ways of coping with this distress are based on defense mechanisms that do not solve the problem, and what is more, they undermine the possibilities for developing and maintaining social ties. Common examples are: Distancing oneself from emotional and social events, and **addiction** to the computer, that places no demands in the emotional field and can be controlled by the user. One of the severe consequences of "emotional blindness," characteristic of adults with ASD, is their sincere desire to communicate alongside their deficient capacity for deciphering the essence of emotional communication. This leads adults with Asperger's (ASD) to develop ineffective interpersonal understandings and strategies, and incites unintentional anger.

The professional literature confirms that adults with ASD are neither calculating nor seek to harm others intentionally. It is most likely their emotional-communicative blocks that prevent the occurrence of emotional reverberation between dialogue partners and lead to coarse and tactless responses, which in turn trigger their failure to connect with others. Additionally, their impaired ability to understand beforehand the consequences of their behavior also contributes to the problematics of this situation.

In order to understand the extent of the difficulty in a lack of communication skills among adults with Asperger's (ASD), let us look at the definitions of the term "emotions" by two experts in this field. Miusik defines emotions as confusing and evasive mixtures that play a central role in the human experience.

Daniel Goleman, in Emotional Intelligence (2007) indicates that emotion is a concept with which psychologists and philosophers have been deliberating and debating for over a century. He suggests that we relate to feelings as the sum total of the emotions and thoughts that are unique to it. He states that there are hundreds of feelings, to which are added variations and nuances, and that far more sophisticated complexities of feelings exist than words can define or express.

An emotional experience includes the feeling at the physiological level (such as a fast pulse), as well as feelings at the conscious level ("Now I feel afraid"). A person with Asperger's (ASD) is unable to express his feelings, because he lacks the ability to sort and formulate what it is he is feeling, which disrupts the mechanism for regulating emotions and is the source of his difficulty in forming empathy toward others and clarifying for himself what he is experiencing.

The adult with Asperger's (ASD) has learned from experience that the way to cope with emotional situations is to physically disconnect himself from them, that is, to step back and enclose himself within his comfort zone. Miusik (2003) presents his version that states that unprocessed emotions "remain in one's body." Phrases such as "stuck in his throat" or "made my blood boil" illustrate the link between body and emotions. Therefore, it is most important that every adult on the spectrum receive professional help that will assist him in examining his feelings, regulating them and communicating them, in the very same way that a mother of a small child intuitively reacts to her child who hasn't yet acquired this skill ("You are angry now because…"; "You're jealous of your sister, but in a minute you'll get a hug too," etc.).

CHAPTER 7

WHAT YOU SEE FROM HERE AND WHAT YOU SEE FROM THERE – ADULTS WITH ASPERGER'S (ASD), THE NEUROTYPICAL SOCIETY AND WHAT LIES BETWEEN THEM

People with Asperger's (ASD) look like everyone else, they do well in their studies and speak their language properly, yet experience the world via logic and clear data. They usually understand facts and statements that have a single meaning. They think along a single channel and prefer repetition and routine over surprises and changes. Wiley (2001).

Lovett (2003), in her book quotes a woman whose partner has Asperger's (ASD), who says: "It's as if we're living in two separate worlds," and quotes another woman with Asperger's (ASD) who states that she doesn't understand "why **they** don't say clearly what they mean." She describes how she sees bodily and facial gestures and hears the various intonations of speech, but is unable to give them any meaning. She compares this phenomenon to dyslexia. Indeed, dyslexic people see the written letters, but are incapable of decoding the words and their meanings. Attwood (in Lovett, 2003) points to the importance of understanding that we are dealing here with two different cultures of thinking and communication.

Where there is a barrier, both those with Asperger's (ASD) and their neurotypical partners pay a substantial price. Their characteristic difficulty in understanding the meanings beyond the words works to the detriment of both sides. In contrast, the understanding that real differences exist between these two ways of communication opens the way to a space that enables creating more efficient interactions.

To illustrate, there is the incident of a young man who successfully worked with a company where he was responsible for their car pool. One day, he discovered a problem with one of the cars and informed his boss that the car must be taken to the garage for repair. His boss asked him to transport some workers before putting the car in the garage. However, the young man was so concerned about the car that he brought it to the garage without having first carried out the workers' transportation. Even though, until then, everyone at work was very pleased with him, he was fired the following day. The company director had never heard of Asperger's (ASD) and in any case was unaware that detailed explanations should have been given to his employee concerning **the reasons** for his request to transport workers prior to bringing the car in for repairs. The young man, however, due to his single-channel way of understanding, acted upon his concern for the car and his devotion to the company. With the help of his supportive family, he finally understood where he had gone wrong, but the damage was already done and he remained unemployed.

The kind old man who walks daily around the neighborhood felt insulted when one of the young boys on the street treated him "as if I was air." He told the boy he was insolent and couldn't understand why his lovely neighbors' son was treating him like that. The old man didn't know that this young boy has Asperger's (ASD) and therefore finds it hard to form eye contact with him and smile at him.

Willey (2001), who has Asperger's (ASD), is the daughter of a father with Asperger's (ASD) and the mother of a daughter with the syndrome. In her book, she describes what goes on deep inside them at interpersonal events. She writes: "You see faces, they become distorted and move. If they are sending you a message, you don't get it... you'll be forced to learn the hard way that **there is more than one message** behind a chain of words, and you will seem stupid, ignorant and ridiculous until you learn that message. You may have to swallow the laughter, the indifference, etc., until you learn the 'normal' game. This is a game in which the rules and expectations of human behavior **have been passed on to the neurotypicals, but not to the adult with Asperger's (ASD.**

I heard a similar authentic description from a dyslexic man. He related how, when he was a child, his parents made every effort to teach him how to read. He would sit with the text in front of him and see the letters floating off the page and flying in the air. He didn't have the tools to explain what he was experiencing, and was reprimanded for being lazy and goofing off. Also adults with the Elusive Asperger's (ASD) suffered criticism from their parents, family, teachers and others in their environment. Like the old man mentioned earlier, it was the same with all the others who came in contact with the young boy with ASD - they were unsuccessful at figuring out how someone as intelligent as he was does not understand the rules of social behavior and makes such tactless mistakes when relating to others.

This attitude gives rise to feelings of social alienation among those with ASD syndrome, and their usual reaction is then withdrawal and seclusion, with some also developing a tendency toward suspiciousness. The fact that, in most cases, they do not understand where they've gone wrong and why they are being blamed, contributes to their desire to seclude themselves. Sometimes there are moments when one will have doubts as to their sanity... trapped in their maze, as Willey writes (2001) She also expresses pain and sadness, when she sees neurotypical people avoiding people with Asperger's (ASD), and intolerable anger at those who make fun of them. She strongly mulls over the question of why the neurotypical population draws away from people with Asperger's (ASD), who yearn for social ties and friendship. The way to understanding and cooperation must be paved for them by their neurotypical partners through openness, flexibility, acceptance and empathy. One mother related what took place when she took her adult son to a doctor. When the doctor was informed that his new patient has Asperger's (ASD), he admitted that he hadn't heard of it before. In his desire to understand this matter, and to learn how to treat this young man in the best way possible, he began to investigate and ask the young man questions about his syndrome. However, this young man failed to understand that the doctor was seeking to learn and to help him. His inability to read the interpersonal map in this situation and his malfunction in pragmatic thinking caused him to react with anger and hurt feelings, creating an unpleasant dialogue.

Literature on the subject confirms what many of these adults and their parents have experienced. At a parents' support group meeting, one of the fathers related how his daughter had gone through superfluous treatment sessions with psychologists. Even though she felt that they were not targeting her problems, she did not have the tools with which to explain what she was feeling. Only after she was formally diagnosed as having Asperger's (ASD), was she able to begin to develop a realistic optimism, with a positive look to the future.

People born with Asperger's (ASD) must survive in a world

that is not programmed for their manner of functioning in the social arena. They may be perceived on the one hand as handicapped, or as people uniquely gifted on the other hand. They are well familiar with the situation where others judge them and criticize their behavior. Stanford (2006) states that it is fair to assume that the greatest damage is caused by the parents' judgmental behavior. In this regard, she emphasizes the importance of presenting the positive aspects of diagnosis for adults with Asperger's (ASD), for the knowledge that others are aware of and confirm their personality strengths can supply such a person with confidence and help him with his syndrome, by discovering his unique talents and experiencing challenges.

Neurotypical people's manner with the world of those diagnosed with Asperger's (ASD) is usually characterized by good will and a lack of understanding. All of us hold prejudiced opinions as to what constitutes "normal behavior." In order to see our way clear emotionally and mentally and treat those with ASD syndrome with empathy, we must neutralize frustrations and anger that arise from short-circuited communication and its consequent behaviorisms. We must keep in mind that an adult with ASD syndrome has had his full share of criticism and especially yearns for positive reinforcement, as long as it is **based on facts!**

Eye contact in a way kindles a feeling of mutual curiosity in partners to a dialogue and builds or strengthens trust. Unfortunately, those in contact with a person with ASD interpret his avoidance of eye contact as indicating detachment, indifference or lack of interest on his part. Because, in the neurotypical society, eye contact is a confirmation of meaningful communication and the creation of connection and trust. In contrast, those diagnosed with Asperger's (ASD), with their basic difficulty in understanding facial expressions and bodily gestures, sense that they won't gain any knowledge from eye contact. They also find it difficult to decipher the significance of a change in one's tone of voice (softness or rigidity, emotional reverberations, etc.). Therefore, their ability to grasp the meaning **beyond** the spoken word is very low, leading them to experience some degree of uncertainty in interpersonal situations.

In the world of neurotypical communication, both a verbal and non-verbal channel are required in order to realize the complete meaning of an event. This understanding raises the hope that with the continuing progress and development of research and treatment of Asperger's (ASD), those diagnosed with ASD will be able to receive help in breaking down more easily the barriers to what is beyond the explicit word.

Songs of the Gorilla Nation is an autobiographical book by Dawn Prince-Hughes (2006), who was diagnosed with Asperger's (ASD) when she was 36 years old. This book presents a personal documentation of her hardships and rehabilitation. She learned to connect with others through the ties she created with the gorillas, whom she describes as gentle, non-threatening creatures who let her look at them and observe them in a way that was inaccessible to her with humans. She says her connection with the gorillas was a lifeline – they lack all prejudice, unlike the neurotypical human society that leaves behind those whose behavior doesn't fit in with the accepted view, and "who look through a glass that is mostly opaque." Prince-Hughes (2006) states that painful memories of past failures and accumulative proof of the inability to fit in continue to be distressing. Adults with ASD need others to confirm their attempts and to relate to them. Her story emphasizes how, at every stage of her life, she was nurtured by the ability of others to accept, contain and confirm her attempts, thus helping her, bit by bit, to "clean" the "opaque glass" and break out onto a new path. She takes us to places and periods in her life when the way her environment treated her was deplorable - like that harsh, unsympathetic teacher who thought that Prince-Hughes was rude, lazy and unpredictable, and in front of the entire class told her she was sending her for evaluation because the teacher suspected she was retarded.

When, finally, a new teacher arrived, everything turned around completely. Dawn Prince-Hughes was rewarded with an understanding of her problems, she received permission to work at her own pace and wasn't forced to play with other children during recess. This wise teacher did not criticize her, and even encouraged her to establish and edit a newspaper, and listened to her philosophical thoughts. Only then did she feel, for the first time, that there is a chance for her not to be alone in this world.

It is easy to see that Dawn Prince-Hughes underwent a reforming experience with her new teacher – which ignited within her the first glimmer of faith in human beings from the neurotypical "camp," and perhaps also helped her in adulthood to connect with and fit into her place of work. She relates that even though at times she had problems with her team at work, as she found it hard to follow consecutive instructions and complete complex tasks, she enjoyed a tolerant attitude from everyone who worked with her and discovered that she was able to converse with them. She also won the encouragement and support of her research supervisor, who recognized her intelligence and her autodidactic abilities. This helped her solidify a picture of what she wanted to do with her life.

Of course, there is no escaping the fact that the clumsy behavior of people with Asperger's (ASD) arouses in those they encounter astonishment, frustration and anger. Stanford (2006) points out that the lack of success in planning and implementing routine tasks arouses anger in their neurotypical partners, especially after they have been let down by the lack of cooperation from them.

The motoric clumsiness affects the adult's self-image while still a child, and causes him to avoid activities that may expose this clumsiness. For example, they will become passive observers of a ball game, thus missing a golden opportunity during their childhood to develop skills in team work and cooperation.

If those surrounding a person with Asperger's (ASD) are unaware of the reason behind his different and unpredictable behavior, and are unable to enlist understanding and empathy, the outcome for that person is bleak. The mindset toward him is usually expressed by criticism, rejection, angry outbursts, etc. Even if these responses derive from good will, they confuse him, decrease his sense of self-worth, discourage him and increase the social "fog" in which he lives. As his uncertainty grows, he clings to his will for self-preservation, which takes the form of stubbornness and inflexibility, which makes it very hard for the people around him, even to the point of aggravating the level of friction between him and them. Such a situation arouses the sensitivity of the adult with the syndrome that may lead to hostile reactions or what may seem to him as hostile reactions, even toward things that were not targeted at him, and all this transforms the social world into something unreachable in his eyes. Through his seclusion and obsessive preoccupation with the subject of his interest, this person creates for himself a safe world that can be controlled and to which he can introduce structure and order and reduce experiencing uncertainty.

Robison (2007), in his autobiographical book, shares with the reader the perceptions he gained from the many hardships he had experienced throughout his life. He claims, justifiably, that Asperger's (ASD) has always existed, but simply managed to "slip under the radar." All his attempts to make friends failed. He used to seclude himself and cry, feeling utterly a failure, humiliated and unable to understand why he isn't liked and what's wrong with him. He wanted simply to disappear, and when his pain increasingly grew he drew into himself. In contrast, machinery did him no harm. The machines challenged him to decipher them, as they didn't hurt his feelings and he felt safe with them. As he relates, he developed an understanding of inanimate objects far more than of people. He researched stones, minerals, dinosaurs, continents, ships, tanks, bulldozers and planes. As an adolescent, he focused on electronics and spent most of his time in the family basement, taking apart and re-assembling machinery. He mentions his sense of control over the machines, without a need for mutual relationships between equals. In his perception, machines do not speak, they are predictable, they don't play tricks on you and they aren't mean. In contrast, he has a hard time reading people, he is incapable of observing and knowing whether or not they like him, or are angry or waiting for him to say something. People have remained a mystery to him.

The difficulty for adults with Asperger's (ASD) to identify their feelings and express them results in botched sharing of experiences with their dialogue partner. Therefore, they refrain from such situations and seclude themselves, even though their need to avoid encountering other people causes them great pain. Robison testifies that he himself never wanted to be alone, and that all those who concluded otherwise were clearly mistaken. Being a creative genius, as others labeled him, was of no help to him in making friends and did not bring him happiness. He relates how, due to his limitations, being alone was one of the most bitter disappointments of his life and escorted him throughout his adulthood. Though his outward appearance was quite normal, his behavior concealed his virtues from others and caused him shame. The burden of Asperger's (ASD) went with him. Adults with Asperger's (ASD) traveled a long and difficult road until they were diagnosed. Many of them testify, both in writing and orally, to the positive effect that the diagnosis had on their lives. Robison (2007) reports that this discovery was an experience that changed his life. Prince-Hughes relates how, at the age of 36, she was diagnosed with Asperger's (ASD) and the fact that she had survived until then was "a miracle." Lacking any help or rehabilitation from the neurotypical society, these two autobiographical writers initiated a self-journey to discover and develop adaptation skills.

Via a precise diagnosis of the syndrome, we are able to free ourselves of the past, as Prince-Hughes states. She relates how her rehabilitation was carried out through her belonging to **a group of people** like her who needed friendship, which is critical to one's sense of well-being, to the awakening of one's potential and individual growth.

Robison (2007) relates how, as he acquired an understanding of the Asperger's (ASD), most of the bad feelings he harbored about himself disappeared and he discovered his unique abilities. Both he and Prince-Hughes tell how, out of their understanding that they are not defective, they were able to understand and define their deficiencies in their human relations skills. Robison

(2007) points out that he discovered his life had been a chain of lost opportunities. His strange communicative style, his neglected outward appearance, his lack of control mechanisms to put a brake on asking direct and insulting questions and his analytic manner that was perceived as a lack of feeling – all these pushed others away from him.

Prince-Hughes shares with us her self-journey to rehabilitation in great detail. She kept a diary that helped her reach a deeper understanding of the causes and their social outcomes. She planned activities and joined a group via which she successfully acquired perceptions and observations of the different parts of her personality. However, the crucial "boundary-breaking" occurred when "I began **explaining to people** why I did what I did," and subsequently discovered that nearly all of them were considerate. She gave up on her desire to act rationally, set out for herself a detailed plan for better adaptation and felt tremendous relief when explaining to others why her behavior was crude, so that they wouldn't take it personally.

Prince-Hughes (2006) taught herself to ask questions, such as "How can I help you?," wave with her hand good-bye in parting and other such gestures. She tries to look directly at the other person and to sense the feelings of others and give them a good feeling through her reactions. She remembers to be gentle and supportive of those around her. Additionally, she has learned to distinguish between what can be changed and what cannot, and feels that she is a bridge to the world, which she calls "normal," for people with the syndrome.

Robison (2007) understood that people who are born with an openness to the outside world can reach far in life, because interpersonal skills are one of the most important factors that predict success. He noticed that as the years passed, he adjusted himself to a more expansive way of thinking. He began making a conscious effort to look people in the eye, to moderate his eccentric responses and to address those close to him in a personal manner. He states how these changes and others significantly altered the manner in which others see him, and that it is much better to live this way. When, after many years, he returned to the neighborhood of his childhood where he had suffered so much, he was received with open arms, much to his surprise. He understood that it was because he had learned how to be friendly, and that simply by knowing "what to say and how to behave" made all the difference. People's warm reception made him feel that he was now free and strengthened his belief in himself. We have pointed out earlier that those who live with Asperger's (ASD) are forced to exist and survive in a world that was not planned for their senses and abilities. Similarly, the neurotypical population is not built to understand what lies behind the different behavior and communication patterns of people with Asperger's (ASD).

In conclusion, it is important that we understand that what we have here are two different cultures of thinking, which produce patterns of inter-communication characterized by naiveté, misunderstandings and points of friction. The difference lies in the way people diagnosed with ASD sense, perceive, interpret and process the social map around them, and their reactions to it. The culture of the neurotypical society is based on flexibility, change, constant development, moving forward, creativity, as well as a person's ability to adjust himself to changing circumstances. This culture demands of its members to perceive efficiently and skillfully every possible detail in a dynamic and developing surrounding.

The culture of self-preservation for adults with Asperger's (ASD) dictates constancy and routine, planning and structure, clear and solid positions and values and unambiguous communication. The source of all these, and more, is to be found in the different functional patterns of the brain, causing the adult with ASD a basic and fundamental difficulty in adjusting to the neurotypical world in which he lives. Since those coping with Asperger's (ASD) have no control over their neurological dysfunction and they are unable to "fix" it, they cling to their need to stick with what is familiar and known to them, and to aim for some control of the situations and relationships which they are part of. The manner in which they perceive the world is logical in their eyes, but does not always fit into the neurotypical society's manner of thinking and behaving, which clearly leads to confrontations. Lovett (2005) explains that the manner in which we perceive the behavior of others is based on our understanding of the situation and the way we react to it. Due to the difference in the brain's functioning between adults with the syndrome and neurotypical adults, **each side is surprised** by the behavior of the other.

Those diagnosed with Asperger's (ASD) are a minority group within the neurotypical culture. They need help in finding ways to adjust, in order to acquire a reasonable degree of independence as adults. Through the improvement of social skills, they will be able to fulfill their aspirations and potential and integrate into society, each in his own way and according to his abilities.

PART II

GROUP FACILITATION WITH THE INTEGRATIVE CBT METHOD (SYNCHRONIZING CONTENT AND PROCESS)

CHAPTER 1

THE EMPOWERING FORCE OF A GROUP –
THE CHOIR AS AN ALLEGORY

A choir is a group of people whose objective is to create a harmonic integration between the voices of all its members. The voice of the individual draws strength from the "togetherness." His motivation is to recruit the very best of his singing talent, and he experiences connection, belonging, cohesiveness and partnership. This makes him feel he is a significant part of the whole, the choir.

The choir has a long way to go until it reaches optimal harmony. Many rehearsals will be held, during which, with the help of the choir master, the choir's work will be interrupted and reviewed again and again to find what went wrong in the synchronization and execution of the music. The process will require perseverance and commitment from everyone. Gradually, a feeling that each one can rely on the other will develop and give his best, and thus a vocal and social harmony will be created. In this manner the empowerment of the individual is developed within the group. In light of the accumulative experience in the field of rehabilitation, there is general agreement that group work is the methodology that significantly helps to achieve rehabilitative goals. It is applicable in different areas of rehabilitation and during its various stages. Group counseling has clear advantages in rehabilitating challenged populations whose members share special needs in common. The support that the individual receives from the group of people who are like him eases the personal and interpersonal tension, in an atmosphere free of stigmas that he encounters in society-at-large and his community. This facilitates positive identification among the group members and helps exit the circle of loneliness, while at the same time discovering abilities and limitations and improving social skills. We can draw this conclusion from an understanding of the reasons, process and results of the social impairment of people with Asperger's (ASD), which is the most prominent problem common to them all. The inability to look beyond the individual perception and understand what is taking place in an interactive situation is a congenital impairment that has many consequences. This fact, in itself, explains why a group framework is needed, which will enable these adults to learn and decipher what is happening in the human environment into which they aspire to integrate.

The group is the venue for a social mini-cosmos, a lab that enables learning in protected conditions. The diversity of participants turns it into a "room of mirrors," enabling them to become more skillful in emotional and communicative reciprocity. The collection of "mirrors" in the room helps the person with the syndrome learn, in alleviating circumstances, how to overcome, partially at least, "mental blindness" and develop reasonable skills in reading the social map.

In other words, via constructive feedback and experiencing interpersonal relationships, the group helps its individual members improve social skills and diminish the feelings of isolation and social alienation, to some degree or another, within the community.

The group experiences presented in this book will be conducted according to the theory and implementation of the integrative CBT method, whose principles are described in the following chapter.

CHAPTER 2

FROM UNCERTAINTY TO COHERENT ORGANIZATION – SYNCHRONIZING CONTENT AND PROCESS IN GROUP FACILITATION THROUGH THE INTEGRATIVE CBT METHOD

The integrative CBT method is a facilitating model, well-anchored in theory, that enables the integrative use of and methodological connection between content and process in group facilitation. This model presents a universal method for utilizing the hidden potential of group processes, in conjunction with the experience of organized learning, while applying built-in protocol techniques. This method is innovative in that it offers a "template" with which any world of content can be planned and adjusted to a variety of populations with different needs.

In the past decades, professional literature has emphasized the need for and reinforced the tendency to a deeper understanding of the reciprocity between the content and the process and development of a group, as well as the need to relate to them as mutually dependent factors whose linkage must be identified.

Integrative CBT is a facilitating method that addresses this challenge and provides an answer. The link connecting the axis of content with the axis of process is the predetermined theme of each group session, with a built-in synchronization of both axes throughout all the stages of the group's development.

The need to develop a facilitating model that is "user-friendly" was identified by the author, following her experience in dynamic group facilitation. It was disturbing to see the increased social uncertainty that was beyond the ability of some of the participants to contain. This was especially blatant in populations that have a unique sensitivity to uncertainty or unfamiliar situations. Vulnerability is especially high among people with special needs, adolescents and people with various hardships in interpersonal communication.

This led to the understanding of a real need to develop an anxiety-decreasing mechanism. The assumption is that through the optimization of the levels of anxiety that emerge in the group process, the risk of anxiety overload will be reduced and the chance for significant learning will increase.

Planning the group and its leadership, based on the principle of anxiety regulation, will enable optimal growth for a wide variety of groups, including populations with special needs. In this manner, adults with Asperger's (ASD) will also benefit from a group experience, which they so badly need. That is because structuring the content and process and incorporating both into an integrative program will increase clarity and a sense of direction for the group members.

This in turn will lead to perceiving the situation as structured, significant and predictable. That is, the participants will gain in the group experience, a feeling of reasonable clarity. This facilitating method is an integrative model for leading groups, which integrates sociodynamic principles with the humanistic approach and is based on perceiving the group as a social microcosm in which the individual grows via the developmental process of the group as a whole. This method applies synchronized coordination between content and process, via the use of themes structured into the comprehensive program, which comprises the group's lifespan throughout its stages of development.

Flexibility is an essential principle in operating the integrative method, in the sense that "every program is a basis for change." The interpersonal dynamics that develop within each group is the variable that determines its state of progress.

The group facilitator has the flexibility to determine when and how to make use of the protocol or the interaction, based on his evaluation of the changing needs of the group. Structuring the content-process relationship provides the optimal viability for the group's development as a whole and for each of its members. It reduces uncertainty, thus contributing to the learning process. In this way, the CBT method can adjust itself to the various goals and needs of different populations, for both the participants and the group facilitators.

The above method was designed and developed by the author with the help of Hava Baruch.

CHAPTER 3

STRATEGIES FOR STRUCTURING CONTENT AND PROCESS AND INTEGRATING THEM INTO A SINGLE ENTITY

The structural strategy of the integrative model consists of four dimensions: The dimension of content, the dimension of process, the dimension of theme (the link that connects the two) and the protocol that integrates the three. In order to understand the role of the theme as the link between the axes of content and process throughout the group's lifespan, it is important to note that the theme is the pattern of an idea that contains within it the topic at hand and its accompanying experiential elements. Instead of identifying the theme from the group narrative, we plan and design it in advance, to serve as a basis for the narrative that will develop in the group sessions. Averbuch (1991) describes the theme as an emotional, experiential and conceptual cluster, linked to every area of content that introduces associative clusters into the group space.

With this method, the title of each session is formulated and phrased in a way that expresses the subject it is intended for, concerning the developmental dilemma the group is addressing and the sub-stage that the particular session represents.

By connecting the two elements, the theme of the session is created, that is to say, the content and the developmental process of the group feed the theme and together become the joint guiding mechanism. Thus, the workshop can be led on a path of reciprocity between the axis of content and the axis of process and facilitate the integral structuring of the content into the process and the synchronization of the two. Through dialogue, the session's narrative becomes cohesive and the theme acquires its experiential-emotional nuances. It is similar to the words (content) and melody (experience) in vocal music, which move between two axes over time and together create a single integrated entity.

The role of the group facilitator is to preserve the optimal level of involvement at the content level and the process level, and to advance either according to the developmental theory principles of the group.

The meaning of the term 'dynamics' is "forces in motion." The forces in motion in a group impact on the interpersonal processes at any given time and along its developmental path. Processes that address the "here and now" are, for example, "Why are we quiet right now?" Processes that address a dilemma related to group maintenance are, for example, 'The significance of confidentiality in the group'.

Group dynamics is characterized by emotional complexity and intensity. To simplify this complexity, we divided the forces within a group into four major categories:

— Social processes (connecting, cohesiveness, confrontation, mutuality, etc.)
— Psychological processes (anxiety, pleasure, internalization, etc.)
— Transference processes – relating to the present (to people or situations) affected by past experiences
— Learning, growth and empowerment processes – the desired outcome of cohesiveness and bonding in the group, and events that encourage change

Social processes – The forces and processes that form and stabilize the social network, maintain it and enable it to operate in a proper and productive manner. These may include differentiation of roles, consolidation of norms, negotiating procedures, advancing leaders, etc.

Psychological processes – The emotional energies that mobilize the behavior of the group and its members. Feelings as the major source of energy of the dynamics, needs, impulses, aspirations, etc., and the emotional development of the group members throughout its lifespan.

Processes of transference – Behaviorisms inappropriate to the "here and now," that emerge from unresolved issues from the "there and then." Transference is a significant and unique mobilizing force, as it raises the need for reality checks and therefore offers the potential for learning and growth. Reciprocal relations in the group are characterized by multiple transferences associated with authority relations, relationships between equals, individual-society relationships, relationships between sub-groups, etc.

Learning, growth and empowerment processes – These are individual-internal processes, therefore the focus is on identifying triggers of learning and growth, as follows:

— Mechanisms related to the framework: Clear goals, suitability to the needs, stability and continuity, clear boundaries, a coherent plan, a skilled leader, etc.
— Mechanisms within the interpersonal space: Cohesiveness,

altruism, interpersonal learning, universality, role-modeling, expanding knowledge, instilling hope and the development of social skills (Yalom, 1985).

A MODEL OF GROUP DEVELOPMENT ACCORDING TO THE INTEGRATIVE CBT METHOD:

This model consists of three main stages and twelve sub-stages. It focuses on interpersonal dilemmas that every group must solve, to then be ready to cope with the dilemmas in the next stage.

Stage A – Connecting and creating a group identity.
Stage B – Individuation via disagreements, confrontations and their resolution.
Stage C – Closeness and mutual connection.

Each group session is a sub-stage along the developmental continuum, and the sub-stages (at least twelve) articulate the tasks each group must complete at each session. Formulating the theme acts as a catalyst for handling the developmental task in each of the sessions.

In Conclusion:
Experts in group facilitation agree that the developmental path in a group's lifespan is parallel to the development (growth) of a human being. It can thus be concluded that the stages of development are universal, predictable and serve as the basis for the workshop's program.

INTERPERSONAL RELATIONSHIPS WITHIN THE GROUP EXPERIENCE

EMOTIONAL
PROCESSES

SOCIAL
PROCESSES

Intuition, Feelings,
Motivation, Impulses,
Trust, Needs, etc.

Normalization, Rules,
Agreements, Roles,
Leadership, etc.

Unresolved experiences
from the past that
are unconsciously
transferred to situations
or people in an event
occurring in the present.

Observation, Interaction,
Self-Discovery, Feedback,
Curiosity, Cohesiveness,
etc.

TRANSFERENCE
PROCESSES

EMPOWERMENT

CHAPTER 4

A MODEL FOR DESIGNING AN INTEGRATIVE FACILITATION PROGRAM

A MODEL FOR DESIGNING AN INTEGRATIVE FACILITATION PROGRAM (CBT/BASIC PRINCIPLES)

The design of a workshop program is based on the work assumptions of this model. Given that the group's developmental processes are universal, the process axis can be planned, with the theme serving as a link between that and the content axis. Each of the sessions is a sub-stage identified by a defined developmental task and suited to the specific topic of that session.

Consequently, themes are created that combine both axes into an interactive program.

THE DEVELOPMENTAL TASKS IN EACH SUB-STAGE (THE PACE WILL BE ADJUSTED TO THE NEEDS OF THE GROUP):

Session	Title of Sub-Stage	Features Of Dilemmas, Issues And Developmental Tasks
First	Connecting	Getting acquainted, defining frameworks, clarifying expectations and a contract of commitment and Confidentiality, reducing vagueness.
Second	Creating a group identity	Deepening mutual acquaintanceship, the process of joining, defining group boundaries (internal and external), an orientation to identify similarities.
Third	Creating a group identity + differentiation	Continued negotiation on the group's identity, moving from the need to find similarities to emphasizing individual differences.
Fourth	Creating confrontations to highlight personal uniqueness	Polarizing viewpoints and positions to highlight personal uniqueness, examining authority relations, conflict, issues of competition and control.
Fifth	Individuation	Examining interpersonal differences, variance and conflict between sub-groups.
Sixth	Resolving the conflict	Moderating the differences in outlooks and positions, through acceptance of the differences and the unique place of each group member

Seventh	Toward bonding	Renewed examination of behavioral norms in close relationships, to create group cohesiveness.
Eighth	Intimacy/Mutuality	Focusing work on personal issues, resulting from the cohesiveness, trust and bonds that were formed.
Ninth	As above	As above
Tenth	As above	As above
Eleventh	Reaching closure	Understanding the essence of personal and interpersonal differences and its applicable significance, and reaching closure on issues toward the end.
Twelfth	Conclusion and parting	Process of separating the private "self" from the collective "self," summarizing the individual growth and learning, and parting from friends and the program.

Session	Issues of The Process	Techniques That Help Addressing The Tasks
First	Reducing vagueness and anxiety	Opening remarks, introducing the facilitators, getting acquainted via a game that gives each participant a chance "to create a space for himself," forming a contract of the framework, and confidentiality
Second	Creating a group identity	Deepening mutual acquaintanceship through a mutual topic, from a general rational discussion to sharing personal experiences and/or an exercise in experiencing, in relation to the group's boundaries.
Third	Moving from the need to be alike to the ability to discover differences	The thematic idea is targeted at examining alternatives in a way that enables agreement or disagreement, suited to the group's pace of progress and readiness.
Fourth	Raising unique patterns and differences, and the development of conflict and its processing.	Polarizing the various aspects of the subject in an "either-or" fashion, to encourage conflict and a bipolar wording of the theme by the facilitator.
Fifth	Individuation (continuing the conflict)	Interpersonal conflict between the members and between sub-groups and the group and facilitator (authority). The facilitator enables the conflict.

Sixth	Moderation of the differences between positions, and acceptance of what is different and unique	The subject is connected to the theme of resolving conflict, reaching decisions and including the variant within the whole, in the form of "both this and that." The facilitator bridges between the process and the content, relying upon the preplanned theme, in the style of "both this and that"
Seventh	Renewed examination of norms related to close relationships.	Connecting between the subject and the idea pertaining to norms of close interpersonal relationships, such as: trust, mutuality, acceptance, support, etc. The facilitator encourages dialogue and illustrates how feedback is given.
Eighth	Adult relationships are examined and learning is acquired via give-and-take	The following themes focus the discussion on the individual aspect, and enable work on resolving dilemmas in the style of mutuality and trust.
Ninth	As above	As above
Tenth	As above	As above
Eleventh	The group members sum up what was learned and turn to applicable solutions.	A theme directed at individual application with the face to the future (in task groups and teams – to achieve mutuality in the practicable work on joint tasks).
Twelfth	Personal leave-taking from the entire group and its members.	Each member's personal summary of what he learned and internalized, and leave-taking via feedback to others as to what he learned from them and about them, so that each one leaves with that which belongs to him.

CHAPTER 5

AN ILLUSTRATION OF THE PROCESS FOR DESIGNING A WORKSHOP PROGRAM

The following is a description of a workshop that was conducted within a rehabilitation framework. To illustrate, we will present the details of planning and designing this workshop, and the process of developing the themes.

BACKGROUND DATA:

The population – Handicapped people who had completed their training and reached the stage of placement at a workplace.

The problem – Diverse and varied attempts (including innovative projects), that were based exclusively on imparting technical skills, achieved the placement objectives in only some of the cases.

The need – In all the above projects there was a complete lack of addressing the emotional needs of the rehabilitant, derived from his coping with changes, which characterize the process of placement at work.

The goal – Achieving an optimal level of absorption and adaptation to the workplace, by strengthening the mental-emotional readiness of the rehabilitant to fit into his workplace, providing personal empowerment and social support during the group activities.

Choosing a name – In considering the needs and the goal, the name chosen was "Toward Employment," as it expresses the stage in which the rehabilitants found themselves and also raises associations such as: readiness, enlistment, expectant changes, hope, etc.

Choosing a central motif - Individual empowerment was chosen as the central motif for the workshop's program because of the importance of addressing the emotional needs, which is critical to successful workplacement in the rehabilitation process.

Planning the order of topics – The order is determined in such a manner that general topics are raised at the beginning of the group's lifespan, and later on they gradually become more and more focused. The model based on this principle is called the "strategy of the inverted triangle," i.e., moving from the wide to the narrow, from the general to the personal. Hence, the order of the twelve topics in this workshop were:

— Getting acquainted and forming a contract
— The handicapped in society
— Joining the workforce
— Responsibility for the condition of the handicapped
— Managing alone or with the help of others
— Routine and changes in life
— Making decisions
— A new workplace
— The limitations of day-to-day life
— The family and the handicap
— Individual responsibility and adjusting to the workplace
— Summing up and parting

THE WORKSHOP'S PROGRAM

The topics listed above were adapted into themes and constituted the program of the workshop's twelve sessions. The program was as follows:

First session: Connecting (getting acquainted, creating a commonality, framework and contract)

Second session: The status of the handicapped person in society in general and in the workforce in particular.

Third session: The advantages and disadvantages of joining the workforce.

Fourth session: To what extent are we, the handicapped, responsible for our social condition?

Fifth session: Are we capable of managing on our own during the rehabilitation process, or must we depend on the help of others?

Sixth session: A change in life – frightening, dangerous or a source of hope?

Seventh session: How each of us reaches decisions in his life in general, and regarding work in particular.

Eighth session: When I enter a new place of work, how would I like others to treat me so that I will feel comfortable?

Ninth session: How do I manage in my day-to-day life with my handicap?

Tenth session: My expectations from my family and my family's expectations from me.

Eleventh session: Individual responsibility, integrating within the workplace and what lies between them.

Twelfth session: Summary of the learning process and taking leave of the group.

THE PROCESS OF DEVELOPING A CENTRAL THEME:

In order to illustrate the process of creating a central theme, we have chosen the topic, "dependency," which is one of the pivotal narratives in the workshop. This topic appears in the second, fourth and ninth sessions of the workshop, which correspondingly represent the first, second and third stages of the group's development.

By way of the title of the session, we illustrate how a merging is created between the specific topic and the specific task of the sub-stage, forming a unique theme for each session. We thus demonstrate how the theme stimulates associative clusters that are meant to impact on advancing the process along its developmental path.

The following is an example of designing the theme for the three sessions chosen:

In the second session, the theme is worded as a topic for rational discussion: "The status of the handicapped person in society in general, and in the workforce in particular," yet it serves the developmental task in two ways:

a. The generality and rationality diminish anxiety. The participants are given a chance to deepen their familiarity with each other in a venue where the threat of exposure is minimal. The topic touches each one of the members and helps to create a commonality.

a. Within the theme, "The status of the handicapped person," lies the question: Who are we? This facilitates the work on the group's identity.

In the fourth session, the theme is worded via the question: "To what degree are we, the handicapped, responsible for our social condition?" The developmental task is to examine strength and influence along with individuation and variance.

The motif, "Responsible for whom?" raises issues regarding dependence-independence, and various positions surface around this debate. There are those who want to preserve the dependency pattern ("I deserve it"), and others who strive for greater independence. There are also those who want to take control of their life, take responsibility and show initiative.

The motif, "Our social condition," may raise feelings of anger, frustration and competitiveness among the group members. This fosters conditions that promote conflict, as expected at this stage in the group's lifespan.

In the ninth session, the theme is worded as a personal question: "How do I manage in my day-to-day life with my handicap?" This enables each member to examine himself with the help of the group. At this session, the tasks of the sub-stage are bonding and mutuality, and the individual can be helped by the group members in examining the sources of the difficulties and identifying resources of strength and ability.

The open question enables each member of the group to touch upon what is important to him. The motif "I manage" invites associative thoughts on functionality, strength and abilities. The motif "With the handicap" raises associations on how one can manage despite his hardships, or how the handicap is a hindrance.

The emphasis placed on the individual contributes to authentic communication within the group and promotes closeness and mutuality. Additionally, individual work is facilitated, which contributes to the mental-emotional readiness of the person in rehabilitation to assimilate into his workplace.

In conclusion, it is noteworthy that this program was implemented with success and its participants (except for one who fell ill) were absorbed and integrated into their workplaces at the end of the workshop.

Part Three presents a program of a series of workshops for developing social life skills, using the integrative CBT method. These workshops were developed in response to the unique needs of adults with Asperger's (ASD), based on the belief that via improved social skills these adults' ability for self-fulfillment will be upgraded in the various fields of life.

PART III

WORKSHOPS FOR DEVELOPING
SOCIAL LIFE SKILLS FOR ADULTS
WITH ASPERGER'S (ASD)

WORKSHOPS FOR DEVELOPING SOCIAL LIFE SKILLS FOR ADULTS WITH ASPERGER'S (ASD)

Positive Thinking Promotes Positive Achievements

I. INTRODUCTION

Upon reaching adulthood, after having left their academic, work or military frameworks, adults with Asperger's (ASD) have a hard time realizing their abilities and aspirations. At this stage, the young adults experience the ever-growing gap between their expectations and their self-fulfillment. They need to cope with frustrations, disappointments and helplessness that are the outcome of their difficulties in adaptation. Therefore importance must be given to every rehabilitative initiative planned and established for them.

Asperger's (ASD) characteristic core symptoms grow out of a limited ability to decipher social situations and, that being the case, training in these skills should be given center stage in every rehabilitative initiative.

The training workshops for developing social life skills evolved in order to address the clear need of this population to acquire tools with which to manage its interpersonal and social relationships. The group training serves as a social lab for learning and acquiring these tools. Inculcating social skills is equivalent to providing life skills. The positive results can upgrade adults with Asperger's (ASD) from a life of survival to a life with development.

The group framework enables its members to cope with their hardships and express their abilities in a variety of interpersonal situations. Belonging to a peer group and the trust created there contribute toward the creation of social ties and increase one's self-confidence. Klin and his colleagues (2000) state that the efforts to develop the skills of the individual together with his peer group must take top priority in every training program promoting social, communication and adaptation skills.

The training method, and the subsequent results as reported by the participants of the groups that we conducted, confirmed that the program and the method are a suitable way of promoting the abilities of these adults to cope with the challenges of life.

BY VIRTUE OF DIAGNOSTICS AND DIAGNOSIS

Adults with Asperger's (ASD) experienced while growing up a confusing interpersonal-social reality. They were repeatedly confronted with criticism of their way of behavior and reactions from their dialogue partners that raised astonishment and deluded both parties. Such interactions and experiences of social rejection caused adults with the syndrome to lose their trustfulness, their confidence and their sense of self-worth. A professional diagnosis enables the adult to undergo a process of self-acceptance. after which he is ready for suitable professional support.

Thus, there is great value and significance to this learning process, as it helps the adult consolidate his self-identity along a reality-compatible track, reduces his discomfort during interaction with others and helps him develop self-confidence. Additionally, he is given the opportunity to discover that he is not alone in his situation and that the community has the ways and means of offering him help.

Lovett (2005) in her book addresses the long-term couple relationships. She notes that when one of the partners is an adult with Asperger's (ASD) who has not been diagnosed, both partners live in parallel worlds and their behavior is different from one another. This situation gives rise to repeated misunderstandings and frustrations. Herein lies the importance of the diagnosis. It allows us to understand and clarify the source of the difficulties, anger and frustration, and opens the way toward repairing and recovering the relationship.

Robison (2007) relates that during his childhood diagnosticians that examined him concluded that he was "lazy, quick to anger and rebellious." Prince-Hughes (2006) claims that when she was diagnosed at the age of 36, she felt as if a miracle had occurred, for up to then, "I was confused because I didn't know what to do in the presence of another person." Meyers (2001) says that adults with the syndrome who internalize their syndrome as a neurological variant, are able to recognize the importance of their skills and perceive themselves as whole.

Therefore the diagnostic process has a moderating effect on negative feelings, both for the person diagnosed and the significant others in his life.

We highly recommend undergoing diagnosis, the results of which will indicate the most suitable treatment program for an adult with Asperger's (ASD), who is a candidate for the rehabilitation program. It is therefore of utmost importance to turn to a diagnostician who has been specially trained in diagnosing and treating adults with Asperger's (ASD). It is worth every bit of the effort!

II. PLANNING AND BUILDING THE INFRASTRUCTURE TO ACHIEVE THE GOALS OF THE WORKSHOP

The rational planning of the workshop is equivalent to investing in the solid infrastructure of any edifice to ensure its stability and efficacy.

The workshops presented in this book will be conducted using the integrative CBT (cognitive behavioral therapy) method. Group development theory will be integrated into these workshops, with reference to interpersonal processes that support the social maintenance of the group (as needed), in the spirit of the humanistic approach.

Workshops for the development of social life skills must be practical and implemental in character. They are meant to address a variety of interpersonal fields in which adults with Asperger's (ASD) encounter difficulties.

The **facilitator** is responsible for the project throughout. This includes:

1. Preparing learning materials for the workshops, summaries, exercises and abstracts for distribution to the participants.
2. Advertising the project via every possible venue – written and electronic.
3. Conducting a personal full-hour interview with each candidate. The interview is titled: "A **Mutual** Acquaintance Meeting." This friendly manner is meant to lessen anxieties at the very first meeting and allow for forming an opinion of each candidate and his suitability.
4. The group must be heterogeneous, yet comparable in age, stage of development and education.
5. The workshops are targeted at adults with Asperger's (ASD)

with a high functional level and the potential for success during rehabilitation.

6. Supportive professional accompaniment is required, including training, consultation and support for each facilitator or pair of facilitators. Additionally, previous training of the facilitators in group work is mandatory.

7. Social skills include an aptitude for the potential bridging between different interest of some group members and the others. The facilitators, whose job is to inculcate these skills, must be of highly developed interpersonal skills together with a social orientation.

8. They must be familiar with the participants of the group they are leading, understand and accept them.

9. Putting a group together is a work of art. The suitability of each candidate must be carefully examined alongside the overall picture of the intended group. People with Asperger's (ASD) have a shared difficulty. Nonetheless, each one has his own individual strengths as well as his unique hardships. The result is that the group contains both homogeneous and heterogeneous elements that contribute toward enriching communication and bonding.

10. It is important that every group have a contract – this will induce a relative degree of certainty and confidence for the participants that they are being guided by people who know how to lead them. There are groups in which the process of building a contract includes both the participants and their facilitators. For groups of people with Asperger's (ASD), the contract is prepared by the facilitator, who then presents it to the group along with a clear explanation of the significance of each of the contract's clauses. A clear and detailed contract

and a well-designed program for the workshop create the feeling of a "safe place" and decrease anxiety, which in turn create from the very start a situation in which the boundaries, rules and norms are clearly understood. This approach is based on understanding the difficulties that adults with Asperger's (ASD) have in deciphering the social map. Therefore their point of entry into social situations demands preparing a solid, clear and supportive framework.

The contract also contains an organizational dimension. It includes issues regarding the viability of the framework, such as: location, time, sequence, detailed program, dates of the sessions, etc. Additionally, there is the social-maintenance dimension. Issues raised for group discussion include: commitment, confidentiality, responsibility, consistent participation, and the hope and belief that working jointly will advance them. The organizational dimension has to be presented as an established fact, whereas it is important that the maintenance dimension be processed.

Protocols of all the sessions in all the workshops will be presented in detail further on, and all were planned in advance according to a predetermined order.

III. TRAINING WORKSHOPS FOR DEVELOPING COMMUNICATION SKILLS AND SOCIAL APTITUDE

The uniqueness of the training workshops lies in the fact that their focus of activity is to address those issues that preoccupy the group members, in order to develop their skills and aptitudes. Adults with Asperger's (ASD) are unequivocally in need of learning through training in the areas of communication and social skills. These skills are acquired intuitively by neurotypical people and develop with age, supported by accumulative **social experiences**. For adults with Asperger's (ASD), training in these fields is an existential need and inculcating it in them is the key to improving their adaptation abilities during the course of their lives.

The training workshop is based on a detailed plan prepared in advance, derived from **what was learned of the special needs of the group members.** The workshop will be based on the information gleaned from the group members, regarding the obstacles that accompany them.

The workshops are conducted using the integrative CBT method, with the activities of each session planned in advance, based on a defined rationale and according to a detailed protocol.

The world of content is the focus of the workshop. The group facilitator guides its members toward adhering to the topic at hand and investing efforts to maintain the relationships within the group. This is an experiential workshop, in which the planned exercise is aimed at encouraging the group to fully examine the agenda-related issues. The facilitator encourages the participants to relate both to themselves and to the others as much as possible, and assists in their learning from the interpersonal ties. This is done within the framework of an organized program for inculcating social skills and abilities.

The facilitator defines the topics, presents the stimuli or exercises and escorts the group's experience, and all in the humanistic spirit. He promotes openness and communication and helps to implement the tasks and achieve the goals.

Baker (2005) asserts that inculcating skills is not "a model of correct behavior," but rather the ideas about behavior that will help the participants achieve their goals. He holds that people with Asperger's (ASD) need, first and foremost, non-judgmental acceptance of their "incorrect" behavior. This is an effective basis for productive work on the processes of change. The aim is to expand the variety of their social skills in order to achieve personal objectives, and not to correct "wrong" behavior.

Most social aptitudes are the result of a mental ability to understand the thoughts and feelings of another person. For people with Asperger's (ASD), the "antennas" that receive emotional and social messages are deficient. Therefore people with ASD are capable of processing the messages only partially and consequently have difficulty understanding the communication's meaning. Usually, they find it hard to understand the point of view of another person, which leads to obstacles in social connections (Frith, 1991; Baron-Cohen et al., 1995).

An aptitude is in fact the efficient use of strategies. Social aptitude is pro-active and has the potential to be of **mutual** benefit. Difficulty in forming ties and maintaining a relationship disrupts the ability to succeed in an intimate relationship, in society and at work. Investing in developing social aptitudes and communication skills is critical to the expansion of behavioral variety in every aspect of life.

Inculcating skills is effective and implementable when it is carried out in an experiential workshop and accompanied by feedback from the facilitators and the group members. Repeated exercises under "work conditions" and day-to-day life, along with positive reinforcements, are essential to the process of acquiring and assimilating the learned skills.

As mentioned earlier, Attwood asserted that for people with Asperger's (ASD), the "land of emotions" is unmapped territory. Prince-Hughes, who has ASD, relates her feeling as if drowning in an ocean that is unpredictable, with no indicative signs or shores. Indeed, it is a very elusive experience.

The workshop for interpersonal communication was developed with the belief that by exploiting the hidden potential of the group as a tool, it is possible to instill and expand the social skills of the participants and advance their situation from that of living a life of self-preservation to a life that continually develops.

FIRST WORKSHOP – DEVELOPING EMOTIONAL COMMUNICATION SKILLS

INTRODUCTION

Both the emotional component and the communication component of Asperger's (ASD) impact on one another and are influenced by one another. The outcome of this mutuality is expressed through the quality of the behavior and social adaptation of people with the syndrome. According to Attwood (2006), one of the major components in social behavior is the communication of emotions and feelings. And for people with Asperger's (ASD), the "land of emotions" is uncharted territory. Brain research done on neuro-developmental perception indicates that the human being is wired for communication. However, when we are engaged in communication of any kind, emotions impact the interpersonal space (Goleman, 2007). For a person with Asperger's (ASD), there is usually a disconnection between what he experiences emotionally and his ability to define and formulate it. Herein lies the need for addressing these issues of feeling-communication-human relationships.

Adults with Asperger's (ASD) have passed through the various stages of development with an ever-increasing avoidance of social experiences. This reaction serves to shield them from painful emotional experiences, such as rejection, frustration and failure in interpersonal contacts. Despite their many and varied abilities and fine level of intelligence, many of them do not succeed in realizing their potential in a career. Thus, upon reaching adulthood, when it is expected of them to build an independent life, their chances for self-realization are obstructed.

The most critical event in every process of learning and growth is the stage or moment in which we understand what it is that we have experienced. In working with adults with Asperger's (ASD), this should be the focus of our efforts, both when working on self-awareness and when imbuing skills and aptitudes.

Up until the latter part of the twentieth century, when the syndrome was first identified and defined, people with Asperger's (ASD) lived among us as "wildflowers" – their different emotional representation was not understood and was perceived as expressing a lack of feeling - due to the absence of emotional gestures. However, in interviews and in books written by adults with the syndrome, we can find repeated testimony to the fact that the emotions indeed exist, but they "are buried deep inside."

Children with Asperger's (ASD) experience failures in interpersonal and emotional communication and repress their feelings in order to avoid being hurt. It is an interesting fact that adults with the syndrome communicate well with children and with pet animals. They express sensitivity and empathy toward them, for in these relationships there is no threat of experiencing failure that ensues from criticism or rejection coming from meaningful others.

The group members' improved ability to understand their own feelings and the feelings of others, along with improved intrapersonal and interpersonal emotional communication, will boost their skills significantly.

The workshop's objective is to recruit the abilities hidden within each of the participants to bridge between feelings and thoughts. The rationale that supports this approach is based on the understanding that adults with Asperger's (ASD) fail in effective interpersonal communication because of the severance between what they feel and experience and their ability to define and formulate it. The current workshop is designed to activate and reinforce the communication between feeling and thought and teach the participants how to identify and define their own feelings and those of other people.

FIRST WORKSHOP –
EMOTIONAL COMMUNICATION SKILLS

Session 1 – Getting Acquainted and Creating a Framework Contract

THE OBJECTIVE:

To neutralize to some extent the participants' **anxiety**, deriving from their sense of alienation in the room and uncertainty as to what is about to take place in the workshop in general, and during the first session in particular.

a. The session begins with the facilitator's opening remarks, which include words of welcome and introducing himself, with emphasis on his educational and professional background. The facilitator then expresses the feelings of uncertainty shared by all the group members in the room, thus showing them that he understands their feelings. He continues to explain briefly that **the basic premise** of the workshop is that each and every one is received as an equal among equals, and with respect for his uniqueness. This is followed by the next stage, in which the facilitator invites each of the participants to introduce himself. In order to encourage participation and openness, he poses leading questions, such as:

1. Your name, when and where you were born.
2. Tell us a bit about your family, your parents, siblings, grandparents, uncles, aunts and cousins.

3. What do you enjoy doing in your free time, etc.

If there are no volunteers for this first introduction, the facilitator invites each one in turn to tell about himself.

He emphasizes that all the questions or only some of them can be answered. During the process of going round the room, the facilitator encourages the participants to ask each other questions and clarify what may not have been understood or perhaps peaked their curiosity. The facilitator's responses are supportive and understanding, so that the questions are not interpreted as investigatory. This also is meant to serve as a model of an accepting and containing approach.

b. The second part of the session is devoted to the topic of **commitment**. Since the sense of commitment is not of deep significance at this early stage of getting acquainted, the focus will be placed on the organizational aspects, such as the framework and schedule.

The facilitator will present the plans and the obligatory conditions that will ensure the participants' success. These conditions include the duration of the workshop, the date and time of each session, etc., as well as **the personal journal** that will accompany the participants at every session. The facilitator will encourage a discussion on the meaning of personal commitment for each group member to attend the workshop and arrive on time for the sessions. Emphasis will be put on the effective learning as a group that will take place, on the condition that everyone attends each session on time: "The cooperation of the members and fulfilling the commitments are critical to our success!"

It is highly recommended that a discussion follow in which each participant expresses his personal commitment, the facilitator should aim toward this and encourage it. The facilitator will then summarize this part of the session, pointing out what the group will experience. He will emphasize that there is no intention at all **to change** the participants. The objective of the sessions is to enable each one to learn how to maximize his abilities in a way that will help him function efficiently in social situations. This objective will be reached via discussions, experiences and keeping a personal journal, both during the sessions and within the framework of tasks to be carried out between sessions.

c. The last part will address the question of expectations. The facilitator will ask of each member to express his expectations. If irrelevant expectations are raised, they will serve as an opportunity for the facilitator to once again clarify and define the current framework, its goals and methods of learning, and to explain why some of the expectations raised are not part of the workshop's goals. For that same reason, it is recommended to write on the board at least one relevant expectation from each of the participants. Finally, the facilitator will present the program's topics for the sessions of the first unit, and the continuity between the units. Additionally, emphasis will be placed on a most important principle, and that is **the confidentiality** of the group. The group members and facilitator commit themselves to keep whatever is said within the group between its members only and at the next meeting, a discussion on this will take place.

At the session's end, the facilitator will hand out to the members a list of the group's phone numbers and a page of tasks.

THE TASK:

1. The facilitator will hand out a contact list with the names and phone numbers of the group members.

2. Each member will contact another member of the group.

3. The aim of this conversation is to become better acquainted, and discover common or different topics of interest.

4. The recipient of the phone call will then initiate a call to another group member, thus creating the continuity of everyone's involvement.

5. In the personal journal, each participant is to write down his impressions from the discussion at the first group session.

FIRST WORKSHOP –
EMOTIONAL COMMUNICATION SKILLS

Session 2 – Deepening the Acquaintance and a Contract of Confidentiality and Commitment

INTRODUCTION

A. The facilitator opens the session with greetings and with **a very brief** summary of the previous session, then asks for a report of the task that was assigned and explains that now they will continue getting better acquainted. He places a basket in the center of the room, filled with items he has prepared in advance (a book, a music disc, a photo album, an interesting painting, a calendar, a vase of flowers, a small kitchen strainer, a clock or watch, a small pillow, a nutcracker, a can opener, a coffee cup, a cellphone, a television remote, a small statuette, scissors, a ruler, etc.).

He then asks each participant to choose one or two items that have some meaning for him. Going round, each participant tells what the item he chose means to him. After everyone has spoken, the facilitator encourages the group members to share a similar or different incident that they experienced, and to address those members whose words they found interesting or aroused their curiosity.

Following that, the facilitator asks the participants to examine the item they are holding and to try to recall a problem they successfully solved or a challenge they successfully met. The facilitator helps each participant clarify which ability, perception or skill has helped him in the past to overcome a hardship. When the participant has finished, he returns the item to the basket and receives feedback from the facilitator. The facilitator should serve as an example and tell something about himself. For example: A kitchen strainer can serve as representing the fact that I carefully strain my words when I want to talk about what I find difficult. It is therefore recommended that the items are such that they can have some significance beyond their practical use. After the rounds are completed, the facilitator asks the group if they have identified similarities, differences or shared topics and what has helped them cope with hardships in the past.

B. THE SECOND PART of the session will deal with **EXPECTATIONS.** The facilitator will begin the discussion about the personal expectations of the participants regarding the workshop. They will be asked to express what it is they would like to improve via help from the workshop and the group, such as: Getting to know new people, learning how to develop a conversation, getting to know myself better, learning how to share, communicate, find friends, learn from the facilitator, etc. By writing their responses on the board, a group "picture" will form. The facilitator will refer to those expectations that will be addressed during the workshop's program, whose aim is to provide tools and skills in the social and interpersonal fields. He will again clarify that the participants' expectations will be addressed via the learning process during the workshop.

C. THE LAST PART will pertain to the matter of **CONFIDENTIALITY,** which is of great importance. The rules that are mandatory for each group member will help everyone feel more at ease and facilitate the group's consolidation. Confidentiality and getting acquainted are the two cornerstones of **THE TRUST** that will be built within the group, and the more the group members learn to rely on one another, the greater the feeling that will allow for openness, which is essential for effective learning. The feeling that the group is a safe place will thus be enhanced.

RULES OF CONFIDENTIALITY: The participants, without exception, **ARE COMMITTED** to never repeat outside of the group what its members related about themselves during the group sessions. Everything that takes place in the group is exclusively the group's "property." You may share with the **PERSON CLOSEST TO YOU** what transpired **WITH YOU ALONE,** and mention the others without noting their names or any identifying details.

SUMMARIZING DISCUSSION: After the facilitator has presented the rules, he briefly reiterates the importance and significance of confidentiality in the group, for the benefit of the learning process, then leads a group discussion in which everyone will participate and be asked for their personal opinion on the issue. The discussion should end with all the participants fully understanding, agreeing and committing themselves. (A reminder should be given regarding the **OBLIGATION** to have a notebook that will serve as a **PERSONAL JOURNAL.** This journal is of **UTMOST IMPORTANCE**, and constitutes a significant link in the learning process).

FIRST WORKSHOP –
EMOTIONAL COMMUNICATION SKILLS

Session 2 – Deepening the Acquaintance and a Contract of Secrecy and Commitment
(For distribution to the group members)

CONFIDENTIALITY – INTRODUCTION

a. Confidentiality and getting acquainted – these are the cornerstones of trust.

b. As the group members learn to rely on one another – openness will increase.

c. Openness and a feeling that the group is a safe place have a positive impact on the quality of learning.

THE RULES OF CONFIDENTIALITY

a. The group members are committed to never discuss outside the group what others have related about themselves.

b. Everything that takes place within the group belongs to the group alone.

c. You may share with a person close to you **only** "what happened to me."

d. In case another group member is mentioned – never mention his name or identifying details about him or others in the group.

THE TASK

a. We meet at the time and place that was determined. **ATTENDANCE IS MANDATORY!**

b. The workshop requires **UNCOMPROMISING** commitment to these sessions. They are a very important part of our program for developing social skills.

c. Try to hold the sessions in a quiet place or at a private home.

d. Each group member brings from home two or three items that hold special significance for him (a memento, a contact, something symbolizing an important event, a hobby, etc.)

e. Each member tells the group why he has chosen the item he brought.

f. The group members are invited to express interest in one another (active listening), ask questions, express empathy with the other's story ("I too had a similar experience") and express their reaction to the story.

g. The session ends with light conversation over a cup of coffee.

FIRST WORKSHOP –
EMOTIONAL COMMUNICATION SKILLS
Session 3 – Developing Awareness of One's Emotions

A. INTRODUCTION

The aim of this workshop is **to open a communication channel** between emotions and thoughts. This session includes activities that will help all of us identify our emotions and distinguish between them. Emotions are transferred from one person to another via verbal and non-verbal communication, 'reading' body language, facial expressions, the eyes, voice and speech patterns of our dialogue partner. It is generally held that it is extremely difficult to identify the emotions of another person if you are unable to identify your own emotions. This session will focus on each one's own emotions, how they are defined and expressed.

EXPERIENCE A

The facilitator will begin this activity with a brief discussion about emotions, defining the concept of emotion (is it at all possible?), and describing the importance of emotional communication. The facilitator leads the discussion (reacts, reflects, explains and shares). Additionally, he encourages the participants to contribute to the discussion and bring examples, and emphasizes the importance of one's awareness of the focal role that emotions play in our personal life and interpersonal contacts, and the ability to distinguish between different emotions via our thoughts.

CLARIFYING THE ESSENCE OF EMOTION

1. **Emotions are the outcome of the personal and interpersonal feelings** that we experience in any situation, they are the "color" of the experience.

2. **During the process of identifying a specific emotion**, there is both a physical and a mental element at play, and in internal dialogue exists between them.

3. **Emotions are private and subjective experiences** that result from both external and internal events (ask for examples).

4. **When the emotional experience is translated into words** (conceptualization) and into non-verbal gestures (facial expressions, body language, etc.), it is possible to communicate it to others. The verbal concept that represents a specific emotion is the "agent" that communicates it.

5. **Emotion is legitimate** even when it is personal and there is no desire or need to communicate it to others. For example: an intimate emotional experience.

6. **Emotion is the energy of the experience** that takes place beyond words. The concept that represents a specific emotion (jealousy, frustration, fondness, satisfaction, etc.) expresses the meaning of the experience in terms of its emotional shades, at the personal and interpersonal levels.

Note: It is important to encourage the group members to contribute to the discussion and give examples. The facilitator must pay attention as to what degree the participants understand the practical significance of emotional communication.

EXPERIENCE B

The atmosphere during the session should be competitive, in order to encourage motivation toward making an effort and investment. Each participant writes down in his notebook a list of concepts that express various emotions (work should be done in pairs). Each participant then reads out loud his list and the group members either approve or reject each item as being either correct or incorrect. It is important to encourage the participants to have a discussion and not feel uncomfortable with differences of opinion. The answers that are considered to be the most accurate are then written on the board. The facilitator guides the discussion and helps the group to determine which answers are the most appropriate.

FIRST WORKSHOP –
EMOTIONAL COMMUNICATION SKILLS

Session 3 – Developing Awareness of One's Emotions
(For distribution to the group members)

INTRODUCTION
CLARIFYING THE ESSENCE OF EMOTION

1. **Emotions are the outcome of the personal and interpersonal feelings** that we experience in any situation, they are the "color" of the experience.

2. **During the process of identifying a specific emotion**, there is both a physical and a mental element at play, and in internal dialogue exists between them.

3. **Emotions are private and subjective experiences** that result from both external and internal events (ask for examples).

4. **When the emotional experience is translated into words** (conceptualization) and into non-verbal gestures (facial expressions, body language, etc.), it is possible to communicate it to others. The verbal concept that represents a specific emotion is the "agent" that communicates it.

5. **Emotion is legitimate** also when it is personal and there is no desire or need to communicate it to others. For example: an intimate emotional experience.

6. **Emotion is the energy of the experience** that takes place beyond words. The concept that represents a specific emotion (jealousy, frustration, fondness, satisfaction, etc.) expresses the meaning of the experience in terms of its emotional shades, at the personal and interpersonal levels.

TASK

a. Meeting as usual, **attendance is mandatory.** Each group member chooses three words, out of a list of pleasant and unpleasant emotions, which represent emotions that are unclear to him.

b. The group discusses their meanings and together form sentences for each of these emotions.

c. The group works together on the additional lists (a + b) and pairing the opposites between the two lists (fear + courage = a pair, respect + disrespect = pair, etc.).

The session ends with light conversation and coffee.

PLEASANT EMOTIONS		
Sympathy	Respect	Confidence
Courage	Excitement	Consolation
Encouragement	Enjoyment	Honesty
Peacefulness	Passion	Admiration
Pleasure	Happiness	Satisfaction
Joy	Acceptance	Amazement
Relief	Pride	Trust
Surprise		

UNPLEASANT EMOTIONS		
Fear	Hatred	Jealousy
Loneliness	Sadness	Despair
Alienation	Overload	Rejection
Opposition	Doubt	Humiliation
Anger	Confusion	Insult
Fury	Deprivation	Confusion
Frustration	Panic	Emptiness
Helplessness	Revulsion	Failure
Loss		

Each participant must himself connect between opposite emotions and compare the results with his fellow group members (as illustrated in the chart).

	LIST A	LIST B
1	Honor	Deprivation
2	Courage	Doubt
3	Trust	Helplessness
4	Discomfort	Forgiveness
5	Hope	Misery
6	Happiness	Frustration
7	Anger	Compassion
8	Passion	Tension
9	Belonging	Pessimism
10	Joy	Rejection
11	Satisfaction	Indifference
12	Admiration	Suspicion
13	Fury	Despair
14	Resourcefulness	Scorn
15	Optimism	Revulsion
16	Sympathy	Suffering
17	Excitement	Contempt
18	Certainty	Release
19	Peacefulness	Amazement
20	Restraint	Sadness
21	Closeness	Panic
22	Enjoyment	Loneliness
23	Satisfaction	Alienation
24	Disappointment	Fear

FIRST WORKSHOP –
EMOTIONAL COMMUNICATION SKILLS

Session 4 – Deepening the Understanding of Emotional Concepts Experientially

INTRODUCTION

Emotion is aroused through external and internal **stimuli** (the armchair is comfortable, it's stuffy in a closed place, it's scary in the dark, a party is happy). We will now delve deeper into these issues and learn how to identify emotions created by internal stimuli (suspiciousness, despair, peacefulness, courage) and external stimuli (the boss is angry – insult, regret, etc.).

EXPERIENCE A – THE CONNECTION BETWEEN WHAT IS SAID AND WHAT IS FELT

We will read the sentences you wrote as your home tasks and discuss the connection between the sentence and the emotion you wrote about.

The facilitator will help internalize the meaning of each emotional concept and through his initiative the following question will be raised: How can we explain the fact that different people experience the same event in different ways? A discussion among the participants should be encouraged.

EXPERIENCE B – UNDERSTANDING EMOTIONS EXPERIENTIALLY

The facilitator explains to the group members that the experience will be personal, after which it will be shared with the group. The members remain in the room and are instructed to shut their eyes, relax and breathe deeply in preparation for the exercise in guided imagery. They are then asked to imagine an event in which they experienced an emotion relating to another person, and are requested to experience it once more. This exercise is done **with eyes shut** and continues for **only** three minutes.

INSTRUCTIONS

Imagine the event, your dialogue partner and how this incident is unfolding, and try to perceive which emotions are surfacing and what are the bodily sensations. We will later discuss this and share with the group.

Everyone shares with the other members the experience he has had, and the facilitator encourages them to ask and clarify those aspects they found interesting, while engaging in an interactive discussion.

THE INFLUENCE OF FACTORS ON EMOTIONS – INTERNAL? EXTERNAL?

Example A: Robert is squirming in pain from a toothache and absolutely refuses to get treatment. What does he feel (fear, anxiety, threat, panic)?

Example B: Jeff's brother fell in battle heroically. What has this caused Jeff to feel (fear, anxiety, depression, sadness, longing, pride, admiration)?

Example C: Abe is a veteran soccer player with a leading soccer team. During the last game, he felt that he no longer has the energy it takes and he is planning to retire. How does this make him feel (uncertainty, sadness, failure, anxiety, depression)?

THE INFLUENCE OF EXTERNAL FACTORS ON EMOTIONS

Environmental factors may have significant influence in shaping our thoughts, beliefs and feelings, as well as one's cultural background, traditions, family beliefs, etc.

Example A: What does an adolescent girl feel, whose ex-boyfriend treated her rudely, when other boys try to get close to her (Thought – boys are violent; Emotion – fear, rejection, suspicion)?

Example B: The daughter wants to play soccer, but her family wants her to study ballet. The son wants to be a dancer, and his family is against it because "he has to be a sportsman." What will the son and daughter feel (Thought – they don't understand me or accept me; Emotion – insult, frustration, anger)?

Example C: Fred is sitting on the sidelines, watching his friends play ball. (Thought – they don't want me because I'm not as fast as they are; Feeling – sadness, rejection, jealousy, frustration).

IN CONCLUSION:

Differentiation should be made between concepts that verbally describe the emotion itself and concepts that describe an emotional state.

An **emotional state** is a concept that describes **a situation** in which someone is undergoing an experience resulting from one or more emotions, which are the outcome of an external or internal event.

FIRST WORKSHOP –
EMOTIONAL COMMUNICATION SKILLS

Session 4 – Deepening the Understanding of Emotional Concepts Experientially

(For distribution to the group members)

INTRODUCTION

1. Emotion is aroused when our internal balance is disrupted.
2. It is the result of external and internal stimuli.
3. For example: A beautiful view – pleasure; a steep decline – fear; achievements – pride; failure – shame; sickness – helplessness; war – concern, etc.
4. Environmental factors may have significant influence in shaping our thoughts, beliefs and feelings, as well as our cultural background, traditions, family beliefs, etc.
5. Differentiation should be made between concepts that verbally describe the emotion itself and concepts that describe an emotional state.
6. An **emotional state** is a concept that **describes** a situation in which someone is undergoing an experience resulting from an external or internal event.

TASK

We meet as usual. **Attendance is mandatory**.

1. Each member writes in his journal three events in which he remembers an emotional state, and at the session he shares

this with the other members. Each member will try to identify how the emotion or emotions experienced should be labeled.

2. Each member gets a list of the **emotional states** and together the group discusses the attached list of concepts. Each one marks those concepts that are unclear to him and asks his fellow participants what they mean.

Acceptance	Leave-Taking	Indifference	Overload
Remoteness	Vulnerability	Listening	Wish
Being Tested	Relinquishment	Pessimism	Ambitiousness
Confrontation	Withdrawal	Evasion	Being Stuck
Optimism	Escape	Impatience	Stubborn
Obligation	Faking	Self-Exposure	Crisis
Nuisance	Being Threatened		

FIRST WORKSHOP –
EMOTIONAL COMMUNICATION SKILLS
Session 5 – The Text and the Context

INTRODUCTION

At a social gathering, a live discussion took place among the participants, in which they shared experiences and exchanged information on a variety of subjects. When it was Gabriel's turn to speak, he chose a subject related to Jewish philosophy that interested him. He went into great detail and repeatedly quoted great biblical scholars. His audience grew tired and expressed their impatience in different ways (shutting their eyes, trying to hint to him that he should change the subject, one person left his seat and others yawned). Gabriel was impervious to all of this and continued lecturing enthusiastically. He was totally immersed in the text and did not discern the context.

A DISCUSSION ON THE RELATIONSHIP BETWEEN TEXT AND CONTEXT

When we find it difficult to decipher the context in which verbal communication takes place, understanding the verbal text in itself is not sufficient in order to gain **an overall perception** of the situation. Thus, the ability to develop effective communication with the dialogue partner is impaired. In such cases, we are often left surprised, uncomprehending and also hurt by the reaction of our dialogue partner. It is clear, therefore, that not understanding the context of a given situation may lead to an

inappropriate reaction. This may be perceived by the dialogue partner or partners as tactlessness, lack of interest, rudeness, cheekiness and strangeness, and may even arouse reactions of anger, rejection and mockery.

What was done ingenuously is perceived at times by others as done intentionally. This can happen at one's place of work, in a social situation or in the family and at times it may lead to losing one's job, losing friends and losing one's self-confidence.

Understanding the context is significant in bonding and connecting with others. One can learn how to be aware of one's surroundings and those around him, to observe, listen and pay attention to the communication codes of the face, body, speech and voice. Increasing the ability to perceive these signals and decipher them forms the basis for an improved quality of one's social life. The following exercises will draw the attention of the participants toward relating to a given situation in full and to the interpersonal context. What takes place beyond the words, from every aspect, will facilitate a better understanding of the communication event and will help those with Asperger's (ASD) participate in interpersonal connections in an appropriate manner.

EXERCISES IN UNDERSTANDING THE CONTEXT AND ITS SIGNIFICANCE

These exercises will encourage the participants to relate to a situation, to its context and also to the consequences and results. It will be carried out by relating to events that happened **in reality**, diagnosing them and examining more effective options.

The facilitator will help the entire group at the session to develop together the appropriate response, via an interactive discussion and brainstorming for each event.

Following is a list of events that will be presented to the group for discussion. Three minutes are allocated to each event for the group members to write their answers in their personal journals.

1. David worked in a large insurance company. He was industrious, effective and well-liked. One day he knocked on the office door of a very senior company executive, to confess his love to her. What took place there? How should it have happened differently? What was the outcome? Describe in detail.

2. The mother of 22-year-old Ruth checked out the price offers for gardening work in her yard. The second gardener whom she called quoted a certain price for 250 plants. When the mother told the gardener that she had had a cheaper offer, Ruth intervened and said: "But the first gardener offered a smaller amount of plants." Where did Ruth go wrong? How could she have reacted differently? Explain and describe what the mother felt.

3. George is a college student. When a new lecturer arrived at the beginning of the semester, George tended to follow him during the breaks. When the lecturer noticed this, he asked: "George, why are you following me?" and George answered, "Because you're new here and I want to get to know you." What would you suggest to George? Give detailed answers.

4. Debbie dreamed of being a pianist one day and spent hours practicing the piano daily, with great determination and commitment. Her older brother, whom she admired as he was considered an excellent student, said to her: "I don't think you play well enough, you'll never be a pianist." What took place here? What was the outcome of this event? How did

Debbie react? Describe what she felt and how she behaved.

5. Daniel, a student of electronic engineering, noticed that the lecturer was "favoring" two of the other students. This seemed unfair to him, so he stood up in the middle of the lesson and in front of the class said to the lecturer: "It's not right that you're always letting them talk, others also raise their hands and want to participate." What happened here? What were the consequences of this event? How did the lecturer respond? Try to describe and imagine the lecturer's response. How would you suggest to Daniel to have acted differently?

6. Donna and Ron went to the movies. As they were standing in line to buy tickets, the girl in front of them suddenly passed out and fell to the floor. One of the men who was standing in line bent over her in order to resuscitate her, and then Donna excitedly said to Ron: "Call the police, he's raping her." What can be learned from this event? What caused Donna to react as she did? What emotions were aroused in her?

7. Mike and Leo shared a student apartment. One morning, Mike asked Leo if he could add one of his shirts to the laundry Leo was loading in the washing-machine. He explained that he's in a rush to go to work and needs the shirt urgently for that evening. Leo refused, and replied that he will not have them live in the apartment like a married couple. What went wrong here? What caused Leo to get confused? How could he have handled himself in a more effective way?

8. Sara and Ann had learned together in school in the same class for many years, but did not meet again since then. One day, they bumped into each other on the street and decided to have a cup of coffee together and catch up on each other's lives. When they were about to part, Sara told Ann that she

is an administrative director of an international hi-tech company, to which Ann responded: "If you're working in an office, you're just a clerk." What do you think Sara felt at that moment? And what do you think she answered in return? Phrase two different and conflicting answers.

9. A young man named Richard was flying to New York to meet his relatives. In line for the security check, he was asked to open his suitcases, but refused to do so and got angry. He claimed that he was an honest person and had never broken the law and therefore there was no reason that he be inspected like that. What is it that Richard didn't understand and that misled him to his reaction? Try to guess as best as you can.

10. Sam completed his university studies and was searching for work. In order to support himself, he meanwhile also worked as a gardener. When he finally was called in for an interview at a hi-tech company, he decided that in order to reach the interview on time and not miss work hours, he would go directly to the company's office without washing up or changing clothes. What were the results of this interview? Why? Try to think of three options.

SUMMARY

The discussion will focus on the following issues:

a. Everyone makes a mistake sometimes, but understanding the situation significantly contributes to decreasing the number and quality of the mistakes. There are several resources of information that should be considered in order to decrease the chances of making a mistake.

b. What do you learn from the stories brought here as examples?

The facilitator will help generate personal perceptions **and encourage the participants to bring their own examples**. The sessions that will follow will deal with how to read people through the help of body language, deciphering codes of speech, voice codes, eye and facial expressions.

FIRST WORKSHOP –
EMOTIONAL COMMUNICATION SKILLS
Session 5 – The Text and the Context
(For distribution to the group members)

TEXT AND CONTEXT

1. When we find it difficult to decipher the context in which verbal communication takes place, understanding the verbal text in itself is not sufficient in order to gain **an overall perception** of the situation.

2. As a result, the ability to develop effective communication with the dialogue partner is impaired.

3. In such cases, we are often left surprised, uncomprehending and also hurt by the reaction of our dialogue partners and we find it hard to respond.

4. Not understanding the context of a given situation may lead to an inappropriate reaction.

5. Such behavior may be perceived by the dialogue partner or partners as tactlessness, lack of interest, rudeness, cheekiness and strangeness, and may even arouse reactions of anger, rejection and mockery.

6. An innocent reaction is often perceived as purposely done and arouses the respondent's objection.

7. This can happen at one's place of work, in a social situation and even in the family.

8. At times it may lead to negative consequences, such as losing one's self-confidence, losing one's job or losing friends.

9. Understanding the context - that is, the place, time and the people (including the relationships between them), being aware of what is taking place around you and absorbing the cues – all these are the basis for improving the quality of one's interpersonal and social life.

10. Everyone makes mistakes at times, but understanding the situation and all its factors significantly contributes to lessening the risks of making a mistake and increases the chances for an effective correction.

11. Remember! Every mistake can be corrected! You can admit to your mistake, understand its consequences, give it some thought and manage rehabilitative communication (admitting the mistake, apologizing, giving a matter-of-fact explanation, consulting with someone who can be of help, etc.).

THE TASK

Each member writes in his journal an event in which he or someone else misunderstood the situation and reacted inappropriately. This event will be brought before the group for discussion.

What is the data of the situation? What wasn't taken into consideration? How could the situation have been better understood? What ways are at our disposal to correct the mistake? Was it possible to consult with someone you rely on?

Share with the group everything you have learned from this experience.

After all the discussions are completed, the group will go to the park or the beach for a picnic. Each member will bring something – food or drink. Someone from the group will coordinate the refreshments.

Be happy, be free, enjoy yourselves!

FIRST WORKSHOP –
EMOTIONAL COMMUNICATION SKILLS
Session 6 – Body Language – Gestures and Mannerisms*

INTRODUCTION

The facilitator's opening remarks: From a developmental aspect, body language is in fact our first language. It serves as a communication tool between an infant and his environment, even before the pre-verbal stage. This is a natural language, for it is direct and immediate. Verbal language, in contrast, allows for thinking, manipulating and even pretending.

In light of all the above-said, clearly investment must be made to improve one's understanding of body language, which will provide greater ability in deciphering the thoughts, intentions and feelings that "color" interpersonal communication. We shall do this with the help of the following experiences:

EXPERIENCE A – IDENTIFYING AND DECIPHERING BODY GESTURES (VIA PHOTOGRAPHS*)

The code of body language is the combination of gestures, movements and mannerisms through which messages are transmitted. From observing them closely, we can learn about the communicators and what they are experiencing and what is happening between them.

The participants receive **photographic pictures** that present different body gestures. Each participant receives one photo and writes in his journal the things he has noticed about the photo and what the person in the photo is experiencing. He then passes the photo to the person to his right, thus until everyone in the group receives all the photos and writes his comments about each photo in his journal. The photos are then placed in the middle of the circle. Each member reads in his turn what he wrote of a particular photo and the reactions are compared for their similarity or difference. This process is repeated and carried out for each of the photos until the rounds are completed.

In conclusion: A discussion is held of what was learned from this exercise. The facilitator observes and encourages making eye contact throughout the exercise. During the discussion of the photos, it is a good idea to project the image under discussion unto a screen or place it on a table in the middle of the circle. (See Appendix of Photos)

Sessions 6-10 were inspired by the book, How To Read People, *by Lillian Glass (2006), Zmora-Bitan Publishers.*

EXPERIENCE B — PERFORMING GESTURES (TRANSMITTING A SOCIAL OR EMOTIONAL MESSAGE WITHOUT SPEAKING)

At this stage, the facilitator demonstrates various gestures (see list below) and the group members write the meaning of these gestures in their journals (what is happening to the person himself and what can be learned of his desires, intentions and feelings). After performing the gestures, the facilitator leads the group discussion to draw out the maximum perceptions from what was demonstrated.

A list of gestures that testify to what is happening to the person as he performs them (the facilitator demonstrates each gesture and the group members decipher it):

1. Folding your arms – you are expressing disagreement, refusal, **frustration and protest.**
2. Your body moves about – you are expressing **impatience, boredom.**
3. Tapping your feet – something **is annoying you**, but you are unable to discuss it.
4. The body is gathered inwardly and closed – you are **overwhelmed with anxieties** in your current situation and are protecting yourself.
5. Shrugging your shoulders and putting out your hands – you **are surprised** and are unable to understand how such a thing could happen.
6. You walk with your head down – you feel **unconfident, despondent and worried** or depressed.
7. Your walk has a spring to it, you hold your head up and your arms are relaxed – you are **proud and happy** about a success or good news.
8. Your arms are placed on your hips – you refuse to fulfill a request or a demand, you are demonstrating your protest.
9. Clenched fists – you are **"exploding with anger,"** which you're keeping locked inside.

EXPERIENCE C – PERFORMING GESTURES DURING INTERACTION

Each group member by turn chooses a partner. Each pair is asked to decide on a topic for a short discussion. They sit or stand (as needed) in the center of the group circle, talk about the topic they have chosen and accompany their discussion with gestures and mannerisms. The group members react to the gestures based on their understanding of the situation.

IN SUMMARY

The facilitator guides the group discussion and calls attention to how body language reinforces verbal messages, but **can also conceal** them, and indicates two or three examples of movements that contradict the verbal message. For example: A non-verbal message – a smiling face and warm attitude; the verbal message –"As of next week, the managers decided you are no longer employed"; a non-verbal message – a solemn, frustrated, unfriendly (jealous) expression and the verbal message – "Well done! You performed brilliantly this evening."

After that, discussion is held on what the partners experienced as they performed the bodily gestures and what they learned about themselves. The facilitator leads toward generating insights.

A list of gestures that exemplify what happens during interaction:

1. Leaning forward toward your partner – listening, paying attention, wanting to understand.
2. Supporting your head with both hands – having passing thoughts or being tired of a situation.
3. Turning your body and face away from your partner – losing interest in the discussion or feeling insulted.
4. Restless hand motions while talking – a resolute desire to convince the other person.
5. Pointing your finger toward another person – expression of placing blame or a threat.

6. Frequent touching of the dialogue partner or exaggerated closeness – an inappropriate way of growing closer.

7. Swinging your feet while talking or listening – intolerance or impatience.

8. Legs positioned forward and wide apart – feeling comfortable.

9. Your head bent downward while in a conversation – embarrassment, hiding a secret or shame.

FIRST WORKSHOP –
EMOTIONAL COMMUNICATION SKILLS

Session 6 – Body Language – Gestures & Mannerisms
(For distribution to the group members)

INTRODUCTION

a. From a developmental aspect, body language is our first language. It is the mechanism that puts into motion communication between an infant and his mother.

b. Body language is authentic, it is direct and immediate.

c. Verbal language enables manipulation and pretending.

d. Politicians are usually considered as gifted in verbal manipulation.

e. Clearly, investment made in expanding one's understanding of body language will provide greater ability in deciphering the thoughts, intentions and feelings of others.

f. The code of body language is a combination of gestures, movements and mannerisms through which messages of the communicant are transmitted, beyond the spoken word.

A list of the gestures that testify to what the person himself is experiencing (a sampling):

1. Folding your arms – you are expressing disagreement, refusal, **frustration and protest.**

2. Your body moves about – you are expressing **impatience, boredom.**

3. Tapping your feet – something **is annoying you**, but you are unable to discuss it.

4. The body is gathered inwardly and closed – you are **overwhelmed with anxieties** in your current situation and are protecting yourself.

5. Shrugging your shoulders and putting out your hands – you **are surprised** and are unable to understand how such a thing could happen.

6. You walk with your head down – you feel **unconfident, despondent and worried** or depressed.

7. Your walk has a spring to it, you hold your head up and your arms are relaxed – you are **proud and happy** about a success or good news.

8. Your arms are placed on your hips – you refuse to fulfill a request or a demand, you are demonstrating your protest.

9. Clenched fists – you are **"exploding with anger,"** which you're keeping locked inside.

A list of gestures that testify to what happens during interaction (a sampling)

1. Leaning forward toward your partner – listening, paying attention, wanting to understand.

2. Supporting your head with both hands – passing thoughts or being tired from a situation.

3. Turning your body and face away from your partner – losing interest in the discussion or feeling insulted.

4. Restless hand motions while talking – a resolute desire to convince the other person.

5. Pointing your finger toward another person – expressing

placing blame or a threat.

6. Frequent touching of the dialogue partner or exaggerated closeness – an inappropriate way of growing closer.

7. Swinging your feet while talking or listening – intolerance or impatience.

8. Legs positioned forward and wide apart – feeling comfortable.

9. Your head bent downward while in a conversation – embarrassment, hiding a secret or shame.

TASK

A meeting is held in a crowded café filled with people. For the next forty-five minutes, the group members observe the people entering and leaving the café, as well as the clients that are seated and are communicating between themselves or with a waiter, etc. The group members note in their journal every bodily gesture they've discerned. **Together,** they try to decipher its meaning and write it down in their journals. They discuss and clarify differences of opinion that have arisen (there's no right or wrong, this isn't mathematics). When the task is completed, they remain in the café to enjoy a cup of coffee and light conversation.

FIRST WORKSHOP –
EMOTIONAL COMMUNICATION SKILLS
Session 7 – Deciphering Speech Patterns

INTRODUCTION

Before delving into this topic, let's make a round and hear about your experiences at the café, which was your task at the previous session.

Verbal communication carries considerable importance in identifying **the pattern** of verbal expression. When there is difficulty in identifying and deciphering speech patterns, we tend to miss the necessary insights. Speech pattern consists of the words spoken and the verbal and non-verbal "leakages" that have to be identified by "reading between the lines." Therefore, it is important to find ways with which we can learn to be attuned to the spoken words while at the same time to what is leaking through them, i.e., to enable an improvement in the ability to understand the (verbal) manifest text along with the hidden message. Thus, we can create a more precise picture of the ongoing conversation, since understanding the cues that are beyond words will improve understanding the thoughts, intentions and feelings of our dialogue partner, and will help us respond appropriately.

Example: The daughter says to her mother: "I wanted to tell you that I love you" in a choked voice and a distorted face as if in pain.

The mother: "I noticed it was hard for you to say that."

The daughter: "Yes, It's very hard for me to say what I feel, but I wanted you to know, so I made the effort."

For discussion: What is the difference between the mother's response and a different response such as "I love you too"?

The facilitator will summarize and add his own insights.

EXPERIENCE A – PRACTICE AND ANALYSIS OF SPEECH PATTERNS

In the center of the room a pile of cards is placed, each card containing a description of a speech pattern that reveals information about the speaker. Each participant chooses a card from the pile, as does the facilitator who then asks for a volunteer to demonstrate with him the speech pattern as the partner who listens and reacts. Following the demonstration, which also includes body language, the group reacts to the facilitator's speech patterns and together try to decipher them. The facilitator then leads and directs the demonstrations of the other pairs, each of whom demonstrates in turn the speech patterns described in the card chosen. Following each demonstration, the group discusses the speech pattern performed and what can be learned from it, beyond its verbal context. The facilitator adds his own perceptions.

A List of the "Leaked" Speech Patterns (sample list)

1. Endless chatter.
2. Jumping from one topic to another.
3. The speaker talking endlessly about himself.
4. Blatant crude and tactless talk.
5. A tendency to lie or "improve on" the truth.
6. Talking that comes across as arrogance.
7. Interrupting the other person while speaking, before he

finished expressing his thoughts.

8. A pattern of speech that is mostly of a complaining nature.

9. A speech pattern that is gossipy, that includes spreading stories about others.

10. The speaker diminishes his own self-worth or that of others.

EXPERIENCE B – APPLYING AND DECIPHERING SPEECH PATTERNS

The participants are divided into pairs and choose a topic for discussion. The topic should be familiar to them and linked to their personal lives.

Each one chooses a certain speech pattern, which he demonstrates while holding a conversation. The facilitator stops them the moment the speech pattern can be identified, and the group reacts and deciphers the pattern that is typical of each of the participants. The demonstrating couple is at the center of the circle, and is replaced by the next couple, and so on.

Concluding Discussion: A discussion regarding each one's personal learning experience.

FIRST WORKSHOP –
EMOTIONAL COMMUNICATION SKILLS
Session 7 – Deciphering Speech Patterns
(For distribution to the group members)

INTRODUCTION

a. Verbal communication expresses the contents of the conversation.

b. Identifying the pattern of the verbal expression is of significant importance.

c. Deciphering the speech patterns provides us with the needed perceptions to maneuver as needed for an appropriate handling of the meeting between two people.

d. The speech pattern consists of the verbal content and the verbal and non-verbal "leakages," which require a reading 'between the lines' in order to understand both the manifest and hidden text.

e. It is important to be attuned to the verbal content, **together with** what is "leaked" in the process.

f. Combining the verbal content and the cues that were leaked will improve the understanding of the speaker's intentions and feelings.

A List of the "Leaked" Speech Patterns (sample list)

1. Endless chatter.
2. Jumping from one topic to another.

3. The speaker talking endlessly about himself.
4. Blatant crude and tactless talk.
5. A tendency to lie or "improve on" the truth.
6. Talking that comes across as arrogance.
7. Interrupting the other person while speaking, before he completed expressing his thoughts.
8. A pattern of speech that is mostly of a complaining nature.
9. A speech pattern that is gossipy, that includes spreading stories about others.
10. The speaker diminishes his own self-worth or that of others.

TASKS

The group members meet and together go to see a movie. **Attendance is mandatory**. One of the group members volunteers to organize and inform the others of the time and meeting place (the early film showing is preferable, thus leaving sufficient time to hold a discussion about the movie in a nearby café.) The movie will be about relationships between people, as per the facilitator's recommendation (not of the genre of thrillers, animation or comedy). The participants will pay attention to the speech patterns and the leaked patterns and will meet after the movie at a café to discuss the movie and the speech patterns they identified.

FIRST WORKSHOP –
EMOTIONAL COMMUNICATION SKILLS
Session 8 – Deciphering the Vocal Code

INTRODUCTION

The session will begin with a short discussion of the movie and what the participants learned about different speech patterns and their significance. There is a direct link between emotions and one's voice. The voice expresses the vitality of the emotion, as well as despondency, despair, anger and frustration. Acquiring an understanding of vocal nuances provides an advantage in interpersonal connections. The voice is a significant barometer of the way people feel about themselves and those around them. The voice is connected to the brain's zone of emotions and is therefore an indicator of the emotions.

The tone of our voice reflects our entire personality, and an unpleasant tone of voice may arouse in others a negative impression and disrupt social success. Therefore it is important to listen to the speaker's voice and glean information with the help of an understanding of the vocal code. This will also be helpful in developing an awareness of the voice of the one who is listening. **Deciphering vocal nuances** can promote one's skills in situations of interpersonal communication.

Experiment A – Listening and Deciphering (The facilitator prepares a text to be read aloud)

The vocal code can be categorized according to: pitch, volume, quality and style. We will use these parameters in order to listen, learn, pay attention, absorb and decipher their meanings.

Each member of the group is given the task of reading aloud a very short passage, prepared by the facilitator, according to the instructions as to the type of voice and category.

The group members listen, respond to what they have heard and the facilitator adds his own perceptions about the vocal code that was demonstrated.

Following is a list of the vocal cues and their significance:

1. The pitch:
   a. **Too high** – This can express a lack of maturity, but also insecurity and tension.
   b. **Too low** - It is pleasant in both genders, yet if it is exaggerated or forced, it is perceived to be phony or unreliable.

2. The volume:
   a. **A voice that is too quiet** – Annoys those who are forced to ask the speaker to raise his voice. Those who tend to speak quietly are not necessarily shy, and are capable of anger and sudden rage. Usually they use the quiet voice in order to express hidden anger, and perhaps also sadness or hesitancy or shyness.
   b. **Using a loud voice** – Expresses a call for attention, and at times also reflects being domineering or bragging. It may also be a sign of anger or impatience.

3. Style and Quality of Voice:

a. **A shaky voice** – Observed with people who are tense and worried, vacillators, afraid to dare. At times a shaky voice also surfaces with people who are controlling their anger.

b. **Vocal assaults** - Incomprehensible vocal outbursts that surprise the listener. They can express exaggerated decisiveness or uncontrollable anger accompanied by tension.

c. **Whining** - People who whine are perceived as lacking awareness of those around them, they come across as complainers. This quality of voice is considered to be annoying and therefore those who whine are often rejected.

d. **A course and rough voice** – Perceived as expressing hooliganism, officiousness, tyranny. Even if people with this voice speak soft words, they don't sound pleasant.

e. **A seductive voice** – Expresses a lack of sincerity, manipulation and at times an attempt to enlist others to one's personal benefit.

f. **Speaking too fast** - Anxiety, nervousness, insecurity. Fast talkers tend to cause others to feel uncomfortable and at times it is hard to follow what they are saying.

g. **Agitated tones** – Often heard from people who tend to argue and blame others. Whoever disagrees with them is mistaken.

h. **A monotonic and lifeless voice** - Perceived as apathetic, distanced, nervous and sad. At times it reflects depression or sadness. Additionally, it can cause misunderstandings as its monotonous tone doesn't transmit the unique significance of the message.

i. **A sweet voice** – Hypocritical, says one thing but means another. It is hard to trust such a person. For example: "You're so cute, it's such a pleasure to be with you. I'll make sure we meet again soon" (There's no need to get in touch, it of course won't happen, because the thoughts were different from what was actually said).

CONCLUSION

The tone and quality of voice don't necessarily reflect a personality with negative attributes, yet the fact that a person has an unpleasant tone of voice may raise a negative impression with some people. A voice filled with vitality expresses the entire spectrum of emotions and makes people listen. Such a voice transmits openness and embeds trust and faith in others, as it represents people who are stable, open and direct. People in the company of those with this quality of voice are drawn to them and feel more optimistic in their presence.

The unpleasant voices, such as too sweet a voice, a coarse and rough voice, a shaky voice, a too quiet voice, a whining voice or a very loud voice, may trigger rejection, opposition, anger, lack of trust, scorn, etc.

Understanding the vocal code can serve as a tool to decipher hidden messages that are beyond the spoken word. Additionally, paying attention to the vocal nuances enables a better identification of the feelings and intentions of the dialogue partner.

FIRST WORKSHOP –
EMOTIONAL COMMUNICATION SKILLS
Session 8 – Deciphering the Vocal Code
(For distribution to the group members)

INTRODUCTION

a. There is a clear connection between emotion and one's voice.

b. The voice expresses the vitality of the emotion, as well as despondency, despair, anger and frustration.

c. The voice is a significant barometer of the way people feel about themselves and the world around them.

d. An unpleasant vocal quality may raise a negative impression and even disrupt a closeness between people.

e. Deciphering the vocal nuances can promote one's abilities when in interpersonal communication situations.

A LIST OF THE VOCAL CUES AND THEIR SIGNIFICANCE

1. The pitch:

a. **Too high** – This can express a lack of maturity, but also insecurity and tension.

b. **Too low** - It is pleasant in both genders, yet if it is exaggerated or forced, it is perceived to be phony or unreliable.

2. The volume:

a. **A voice that is too quiet** – Annoys those who are forced to ask the speaker to raise his voice. Those who tend to speak quietly are not necessarily shy, and are capable of anger and sudden rage. Usually they use the quiet voice in order to express hidden anger, and perhaps also sadness or hesitancy or shyness.

b. **Using a loud voice** – Expresses a call for attention, and at times also reflects being domineering or bragging. It may also be a sign of anger or impatience.

3. Style and Quality of Voice:

a. **A shaky voice** – Observed with people who are tense and worried, vacillators, afraid to dare. At times a shaky voice also surfaces with people who are controlling their anger.

b. **Vocal assaults** - Incomprehensible vocal outbursts that surprise the listener. They can express exaggerated decisiveness or uncontrollable anger accompanied by tension.

c. **Whining** - People who whine are perceived as lacking awareness of those around them, they come across as complainers. This quality of voice is considered to be annoying and therefore those who whine are often rejected.

d. **A course and rough voice** – Perceived as expressing hooliganism, officiousness, tyranny. Even if people with this voice speak soft words, they don't sound pleasant.

e. **A seductive voice** – Expresses a lack of sincerity, manipulation and at times an attempt to enlist others to one's personal benefit.

f. **Speaking too fast** - Anxiety, nervousness, insecurity. Fast talkers tend to cause others to feel uncomfortable and at times it is hard to follow what they are saying.

g. **Agitated tones** – Often heard from people who tend to argue and blame others. Whoever disagrees with them is mistaken.

h. **A monotonic and lifeless voice** - Perceived as apathetic, distanced, nervous and sad. At times it reflects depression or sadness. Additionally, it can cause misunderstandings as its monotonous tone doesn't transmit the unique significance of the message.

i. **A sweet voice** – Hypocritical, says one thing but means another. It is hard to trust such a person. For example: "You're so cute, it's such a pleasure to be with you. I'll make sure we meet again soon" (There's no need to get in touch, it of course won't happen, because the thoughts were different from what was actually said).

CONCLUSION

a. The tone and quality of voice don't necessarily reflect a personality with negative attributes.

b. The quality of the voice may create a negative impression.

c. A voice filled with vitality expresses the entire spectrum of emotions and makes people listen.

d. Such a voice transmits openness and embeds trust and faith in others, as it represents stability, sincerity, integrity and optimism.

e. Unpleasant voices (see the list of vocal cues) may trigger rejection, opposition, anger, lack of trust, scorn, etc.

f. Deciphering the vocal code can serve as a tool to decipher hidden messages that are beyond the spoken word and helps identify the feelings and intentions of the dialogue partner.

THE TASK

The session is held as usual. **Participation is mandatory**. The group meets in one of the homes as coordinated with the hosting member. Together the group rehearses and each member performs all the cues. Following each demonstration, the group members react to it as follows:

a. How did the quality of voice and style sound?
b. What emotional response did the voice (not the content) raise in you?
c. What can be learned about the speaker from his vocal performance?

The session ends with light conversation over a cup of coffee.

FIRST WORKSHOP –
EMOTIONAL COMMUNICATION SKILLS
Session 9 – The Eyes: The Spotlights of the Face

INTRODUCTION

Today we will start with a very brief review of what we have done until now. In fact, the objective of the first unit is to impart the foundations for developing skills of efficient communication between people.

The basis for this is the ability to sense, understand and also formulate for ourselves what is happening to the person we are communicating with, our dialogue partner, beyond the spoken words. We are gradually exposing all the elements that create the emotional and non-verbal experience – in order to impart the skills and tools that will help decipher the experience that develops during an interaction, beyond the verbal dialogue.

We began with creating an awareness of emotions and deepening the understanding of emotional concepts in an experiential way. We then turned the spotlight toward the text and context of communication, with emphasis placed on the importance of the verbal dialogue and the context in which it takes place. From here, we gradually identified the elements of non-verbal communication: body language (including gestures and mannerisms), the code of speech, the vocal code, etc.

Today we will concentrate on the eyes - they are the spotlights of the face and the soul. It is noteworthy that the eyes are an organ that both absorbs sights while at the same time reflects our emotions and experiences. Therefore they have a **significant** contribution to understanding other people. In summary, it can be said that the eyes are the spotlight **that projects our inner feelings and emotions outwardly** – they convey to us the essence of what a person is experiencing. The difficulty that adults with Asperger's (ASD) have in forming eye contact demonstrates their communication problems in everyday life.

EXPERIENCE A – A MEETING OF THE EYES

INTRODUCTION: What happens when it is difficult to make eye contact? When was the last time you looked directly at the person you were talking to? How difficult it is at times **to look directly at the eyes** of another person, and if we pay attention to this, how beneficial will it be in helping us **understand** what the person facing us feels and means?

Improving these skills, by learning the codes of reading the eyes, can significantly help in interpersonal communication. Herein lies the critical importance of a meeting of the eyes as a basis for meaningful communication.

The group is asked to divide up into pairs, who will sit one opposite the other. The exercise is non-verbal. The participants are asked to look into each other's eyes, and thus remain for as long as they can. Whoever succeeds in maintaining his gaze longer, will encourage his partner to gaze back into his eyes. The facilitator clocks three minutes and then asks the pairs to switch partners and repeat the exercise. If the group is small, then all the members can practice opposite all the other members. With a large group, the exercise should be repeated with different partners not more than four times. The exercise is then summarized with the entire group, discussing the experience they had, the degree of difficulty, with whom they found the exercise easier or harder, their concerns before they began and how they felt afterward. The participants are asked to report before the entire group what they were able to understand about their partners by focusing exclusively on the eyes (intentions, feelings, mood).

Concluding discussion: A meeting of the eyes is indeed the foundation-stone of communication, and it demands recruitment and motivation. Acquiring awareness and better control of this is critical to improving one's communication. The daily practice of a meeting of the eyes will eventually turn this into habitual behavior, even to the point of being carried out automatically.

EXPERIENCE B – EXPRESSIONS OF THE EYES
The following is a code list of eye expressions (a sample list for exercise purposes):

1. **Smiling eyes** - An experience of pleasant and satisfying emotions, such as fondness for others, a sense of accomplishment
2. **A steady gaze** – Feeling relaxed and comfortable, with presence and listening
3. **A staring gaze** - Aggression, invasiveness, anger, revenge, blame or punishment
4. **Downcast eyes** - Shame, embarrassment, sadness
5. **A deep, direct gaze** – Anger, frustration, disappointment, threat
6. **Raised, staring eyes and raised eyebrows** – amazement, surprise
7. **Squinting eyes and raised eyebrows** - Skepticism, uncertainty
8. **Blinking eyes** – Insecurity, anxiousness, embarrassment

9. **Looking slantwise at the dialogue partner** - Avoidance, lack of trust, suspicion, secrecy

At the start of each exercise, the facilitator reads aloud each code and asks the participants **to demonstrate it** while listening to him. The group is then divided into pairs and the facilitator invites each pair in turn to practice one of the sample codes from the above list before the entire group. This is done with the help of a small vignette matched to each code from the list. The facilitator distributes the instructions to each pair for their exercise and encourages them in their role-play. During the exercise, one partner demonstrates the expression of the eyes and the other partner responds with feedback, telling him what his eyes expressed, what he absorbed and understood from it. Immediately following, they switch their role-play. When all the pairs of participants have completed exercising the eye codes, a short discussion is held to summarize what was learned.

The following is a list of the brief vignettes for the role plays, which the facilitator will distribute to the pairs according to the above code list (each participant receives the list that was prepared in advance by the facilitator):

1. Imagine you are about to meet a person whom you like very much and haven't seen in a long time. (1)
2. You are having a conversation with your grandmother and grandfather, who love and admire you very much. (2)
3. You happen to meet on the street someone who used to harass you when you were a child, and he asks you cynically, "So what's new?" (5)

4. Your manager at work calls you in for a talk and informs you that it was decided to transfer you to a position that is of lower status than your current position, which you love. (6)

5. You find out that a friend of yours at work, whom you've always helped solve complex problems on the job, complained that you work too slowly and therefore you were demoted. What look will he get from you when you meet face to face? (9)

6. You discover the surprise that your family and friends have planned for your birthday. (6)

7. You are offered a job that is boring but with much higher pay than what you've been offered until now. (7)

8. As you are walking down the street, you are approached by a derelict, who tells you that he has no money for food. He seems strange and you are trying to figure him out and decide what to do. (7)

9. You are invited to a party and shortly after you've arrived, you are approached by a young man/woman who initiates a conversation with you and shows interest in you. (8)

10. You are late for an appointment at work that was very important to you. (4)

SUMMARY

The entire group clarifies what its members experienced and learned. What did they find difficult? What was easy? What was clear? What was confusing?

It is important that the facilitator point out that there are no right or wrong answers. The impressions of the observers can be varied, **on condition** that they are relevant to the context of the session.

FIRST WORKSHOP –
EMOTIONAL COMMUNICATION SKILLS
Session 9 – The Eyes –Spotlights of the Face
(For distribution to the group members)

a. The eyes are an organ that absorbs sights and at the same time reflects our emotions and experiences.

b. The eyes have a significant contribution to understanding other people, as they reflect our emotions.

c. The ability to look directly at someone, focus one's attention and decipher the codes of the eyes' expressions helps improve our insights about others.

d. By reading the eyes, we are able to understand what the person standing opposite us is feeling.

e. Deciphering the codes of the eyes' expressions significantly helps improve the quality of interpersonal communication.

A CODE LIST OF EYE EXPRESSIONS

1. **Smiling eyes** - An experience of pleasant and satisfying emotions, such as fondness for others, a sense of accomplishment.

2. **A steady gaze** – Feeling relaxed and comfortable, with presence and listening.

3. **A staring gaze** - Aggression, invasiveness, anger, revenge, blame or punishment.

4. **Downcast eyes** - Shame, embarrassment, sadness.

5. **A deep, direct gaze** – Anger, frustration, disappointment, threat.

6. **Raised, staring eyes and raised eyebrows** – amazement, surprise.
7. **Squinting eyes and raised eyebrows** - Skepticism, uncertainty.
8. **Blinking eyes** – Insecurity, anxiousness, embarrassment.
9. **Looking slantwise at the dialogue partner** - Avoidance, lack of trust, suspicion, secrecy.

THE TASK

The session is held at the home of a group member. **Attendance is mandatory.**

a. The group receives an envelope with photos inside. The photos are placed in the center of the table and each person in turn chooses one photo, carefully looks at **the expression of the eyes** and writes down what he can learn from the image in the photo – what is that person experiencing? What is he or she feeling? What is he or she thinking?

   After three minutes, a round of the entire group is made. Each member in his turn places his photo in the center of the table and the other group members look at it and add their comments as to what can be gleaned from the photo (thoughts, feelings, intentions).

b. The group watches television, but without the sound, and from time to time they pause on an interesting frame (it can be from any program or commercial) and analyze the expression of the eyes.

   The session ends with light conversation over a cup of coffee.

FIRST WORKSHOP –
EMOTIONAL COMMUNICATION SKILLS
Session 10 – The Face – Mirror of the Soul

INTRODUCTION

The main character of the book, *The Curious Incident of the Dog in the Night-Time* (Mark Haddon, 2003), describes how difficult it is to communicate verbally without understanding facial expressions. He explains that people are confusing when they say a lot of things without using words and use their body language instead.

a. Verbal communication is the major means of transmitting information and content to others.

b. The ability to understand facial expressions and decipher their meaning is an important condition for creating personal contact and connecting with conversational partners.

c. Listening and observing facial expressions are the key to identifying the emotions and intentions of others.

d. Listening and observing improve the understanding of hidden messages and social codes.

e. Such an understanding impacts upon the effectiveness of social functioning.

f. The four stages of reading the social codes are:

* Observing the facial expressions.
* Assimilating and deciphering what was absorbed.
* Understanding the significance of the above.
* Choosing the appropriate response.

g. Understanding most of the non-verbal cues of the face and eyes is the means toward identifying the congruency between the manner of standing, sitting, walking and body posture to the facial expression.

h. All of this progressively validates the facial cues.

i. Since the body reacts immediately and instinctively, it tells us what verbal communication may camouflage.

EXPERIENCE A - DECIPHERING FACIAL EXPRESSIONS (FOREHEAD, LIPS AND EYES)

This process in this exercise is similar to a card game. In the center of the table a pile of photos is placed, which are of various facial expressions. Each participant draws a photo, looks at it and writes in his journal:

a. What is the person in the photograph feeling and thinking?

b. What does the facial expression in the photograph make me feel, think, understand and react?

The photograph that each member draws is passed around from one to another, and everyone writes in his journal his reaction to each of the photographs. Following this, a discussion is held comparing the different reactions and interpretations of all the photographs. The facilitator adds his own insights and provides feedback to the group on the work process.

The **concluding** discussion focuses on issues such as: What have I learned from this exercise, where was I stuck, where can I apply this in my daily life?

EXPERIENCE B – EXPERIMENTING IN CARRYING OUT FACIAL EXPRESSIONS

The facilitator prepares notes for exercising facial expressions. The exercise includes two rounds, wherein at every round each of the participants receives one note with an example of a facial expression code. The note includes a short description of a situation that arouses the expression of emotions in the face and body language. For example:

1. You are waiting for your girlfriend in the street, but she doesn't arrive. What will your face and body movements express?
2. You received an evaluation report with especially high grades. How will you react, beyond the words? Express your feelings via facial expressions, without words.

Each person in turn demonstrates before the entire group the code he received, and the other members write in their journals remarks, impressions and feelings. At this stage, each one reacts to the demonstrator's performance as follows:

a. What I think you wanted to express.
b. How did it affect me, how did I feel, how did I react inwardly?

After all the participants have reacted, the demonstrator will report what and how he felt, and whether the other members' reactions indicate that they understood his thoughts, intentions and feelings.

SUMMARY

The objective of seeking out the greater part of the non-verbal cues and signs of the hands and face is to identify the congruency between them and the manner of standing, sitting, walking, the position of the shoulders and the posture of the entire body.

The link between the different cues **makes it easier** for us to understand what our dialogue partner is experiencing.

Remember, the body reacts intuitively while the verbal language enables one to change, camouflage or blur the true intentions and thoughts of the speaker.

FIRST WORKSHOP –
EMOTIONAL COMMUNICATION SKILLS

Session 10 – The Face – The Mirror of the Soul
(For distribution to the group members)

INTRODUCTION
Codes that can help us decipher facial expressions (sample list)

Each participant writes down his interpretation for each of the codes on the list.

THE CODES (A SAMPLE)

1. Nodding – agreement, understanding, empathy
2. Frequently diverting your eyes from your dialogue partner – embarrassment, emotional detachment, impatience
3. A soft and natural gaze at the dialogue partner
4. Looking from the side instead of looking directly
5. Yawning frequently during the conversation
6. A tense and false smile
7. Massaging your mouth with your hand
8. Biting your lips
9. Blushing
10. A distant, sealed look
11. Raised eyebrows and eyes wide open
12. Gazing downwards with lowered head
13. A sad, lifeless look
14. A surprised look
15. A mocking expression
16. A smile at the corner of the mouth

INTERPRETATIONS TO CHOOSE FROM (A SAMPLE)

Fright, emotional detachment, impatience, despondency, shame, surprise, amazement, regret, concern, approval, suspiciousness, distrust, fondness, relaxation, embarrassment, boredom, tiredness, dishonesty.

THE TASK

Each participant collects ten pictures with facial expressions of any kind, from the family albums, newspapers, etc. He chooses pictures that have a challenging facial expression. After numbering each picture, he writes in his journal according to the numbers, what can be learned **from the facial expression** of the image in each picture.

The second part of the exercise will be based on facial expressions from pictures on the internet. Each participant will search the internet and choose ten pictures of faces with interesting and challenging expressions. He will try to describe them and write what he thinks the image in the picture is experiencing, and what his facial expression indicates.

EXAMPLE – PICTURE 1

A middle-aged woman is looking directly ahead with her mouth wide open. Is she calling out to someone? Has she been frightened by someone or something? How can we know? I looked for a moment and saw in her eyes that she sees something alarming or frightening and I understood that that's why her two hands are placed on her cheeks. This led me to understand that she is frightened or worried, as she is witnessing a scary event.

In this manner, the participant is to write in his journal about each picture.

The group meets at a café. Each one brings the ten pictures he collected and everyone together deciphers them. Following that, it is time to celebrate the end of the first unit by going together to a movie. The facilitator will propose a movie that is near the café and will coordinate the hours for the different parts of the meeting. **Attendance is mandatory.**

SESSION 11 – OPEN MEETING TO COMPLETE EXERCISES & ISSUES

SESSION 12 – SUMMARIZING DISCUSSION & INTEGRATION OF THE MATERIAL

SECOND WORKSHOP –
DEVELOPING INTERPERSONAL COMMUNICATION SKILLS

*"Perhaps I made a mistake, every person makes
a mistake or will do so in the future"*
David Ben-Gurion

INTRODUCTION

This workshop steers the group members significantly forward toward acquiring social skills, with emphasis on management and communication in interpersonal relationships.

The first workshop, which focused on skills in emotional communication, exposed the participants to a process of acquainting them with the emotional world. Various means were applied and included a discussion on emotions, different experiential experimentations to deepen the understanding of emotional concepts, exercises in identifying emotions and discerning the difference between emotion-eliciting stimuli derived from external and internal factors. The second part of the first workshop dealt with "communication beyond the spoken word."

Via these workshop sessions, the participants were exposed to the elements of non-verbal communication that are important and significant in creating ties with other people. Thus, they acquired tools to help them draw closer to others and facilitate fostering reciprocal relationships.

These skills will serve as a substantial basis in their work on developing interpersonal communication skills in the current workshop. The insights and skills acquired thus far will benefit the participants with Asperger's (ASD) in creating dialogues and interpersonal communication, and contribute to their effective coping with situations of interpersonal relations.

SECOND WORKSHOP –
DEVELOPING INTERPERSONAL COMMUNICATION SKILLS
Session 1 – Active Listening

INTRODUCTION

This workshop will focus on nurturing communication skills between one person to another, which serve as the basis for all human relationships.

Active listening - Listening that is accompanied by **focusing one's attention** on what the dialogue partner is saying. It is a cue with which we signal our dialogue partner that we are truly interested in him. In a state of active listening, we enlist nearly all our senses, especially our sense of sight and hearing. We utilize them to observe body language and facial expressions, and to listen to voice intonations and style of speech. Listening to the content alone may help to develop a dialogue that relates to the verbal messages, yet with **active listening**, we are expressing **interest in the person himself** and a desire to connect with him and understand him. Through active listening, we increase our motivation to learn about the person facing us and our readiness to apply our senses in order to understand him. Observation and listening are **a mandatory requirement** toward creating **significant** communication between people.

Complaints are often heard of people who "are listening without hearing," but there are also those who hear without listening. The ability to be aware of one's body language helps us absorb through our senses a deeper meaning, as the verbal conversation unfolds. It helps us listen to what the other person **is feeling**, what he **is thinking,** as well as **what he means**. If we can signal to our dialogue partner that we have interest in him, we will be endowing him with confidence and he will respond with cooperation. In contrast, superficial listening expressed through a lack of interest may lead to his diminished involvement and even to **distancing himself.**

EXPERIENCE A (Each pair performs the exercise before the group, whose members observe and provide feedback following each turn)

Each participant performs in turn two roles – that of the speaker and that of the listener – with the partners of each pair switching roles at each turn. To begin, the first participant relates something personal about himself, as extensively as possible. It can be about his life, something from his childhood, his army service, university studies or professional milieu, or perhaps a hobby, or some other area. The listener sits opposite him as the other group members observe them both. The observers write down their impressions of how each of the two role-players – the speaker and the listener – have performed. If some difficulty arises, the listener should encourage the speaker to feel comfortable and continue relating his story. Following this, the two members of the pair switch roles. When all the turns have been completed, all the members of the group return to the full forum and share their experiences.

CONCLUSION

Each participant relates how he **experienced** his role as a speaker, a listener and an observer. He then tells the group what he **observed** of the speaker and the listener. The facilitator will take an active part in helping the participants with their wording, clarification, interpretations and suggestions for improvement. It is important that all the participants express themselves at all stages of the experience and in all the roles.

SECOND WORKSHOP –
DEVELOPING INTERPERSONAL COMMUNICATION SKILLS
Session 1 – Active Listening
(For distribution to the group members)

WHAT IS ACTIVE LISTENING?

- Active listening enables one not just to listen to the other person, but also to give him the feeling that we are with him, by responding to what he is saying.
- By doing so, we are signaling to our dialogue partner that we are taking an interest in him and want to understand him.
- If we signal our dialogue partner that we are showing interest in him, he will put his trust in us and respond by cooperating.
- We can then express either agreement or disagreement, support, encouragement, etc.

IN ORDER TO DO SO:

- When we focus our attention on what our dialogue partner is saying, we must enlist our senses.
- We have to observe his body language and facial expressions, and listen to the voice intonations and style of speech.

Remember!

Observation ≠ seeing

Listening ≠ hearing

- Listening along with seeing and hearing - these are the mandatory preconditions for creating significant communication between people.

- Superficial listening, expressed via a lack of interest or pretending, will lead the speaker to decreased motivation and distancing.

THE TASK – PARTICIPATION IS MANDATORY.

The group meets at the home of one of the group members, providing a more personal ambiance. Each member in turn tells about himself, whatever may help his fellow group members to get to know him better.

The listeners practice active listening: They enlist their senses to understand the body language, observe the face and the eyes and express interest.

After each group member in his turn relates something about himself, he receives feedback from all the other members.

The meeting ends with light conversation over a cup of coffee.

SECOND WORKSHOP –
DEVELOPING INTERPERSONAL COMMUNICATION SKILLS
Session 2 – Handling the Conversation

INTRODUCTION

We will begin with a short discussion of the tasks from last week. The topic today – how to handle a conversation.

Conversation is a central tool in creating communication, building and maintaining connections, as well as deepening familiarity and mutual closeness. Therefore, learning the rules of how to handle a conversation and practicing them are of invaluable importance. This includes all the stages, from the initial encounter to parting. Our experience in handling a conversation enables us to examine our own behavior and responses toward our dialogue partner throughout all its stages. It is an opportunity to raise our awareness of how we function in our relation to others.

The objective of a conversation is to create a connection with another person and exchange with him information and ideas, and make our dialogue partner feel that he matters to us. This feeling will in turn encourage a friendly atmosphere. Accumulative experience in handling conversations promotes our own self-confidence and lessens our fear of failure. We learn how to prepare ourselves for formal conversations, and also how to enjoy light talk. Gradually, we free ourselves from the fear that our reactions will be socially inappropriate, and we become free to utilize our thinking skills. The leading principles in this regard include, inter alia, the use of language appropriate to the situation and the person, and a true desire to talk to people in general, and with our dialogue partner in particular.

EXPERIENCE A – CHOOSING A THEME

For the facilitator: This experimentation begins with brainstorming, in which all the group members suggest various topics, which the facilitator writes on the board, phrased as a theme in order to raise interest and charge the air with positive motivation. For example: Instead of "Global Warming," suggest: "How does global warming impact on our lives today and on future generations?" Another example: Instead of "People and Dogs," suggest: "Is the friendship between two people different from the friendship between a person and his dog?" This style of phrasing opens opportunities for a prolonged discussion that is also richer in ideas. The facilitator will suggest five social and interpersonal themes to be discussed by the group membership.

EXPERIENCE B – HANDLING A CONVERSATION

The group is divided into pairs, each pair chooses a theme. The facilitator instructs them to begin their conversation from the moment they enter the room and their first encounter and up to the parting conclusion. The conversation is carried out in front of the other group members, who observe them and write down their comments in their journals. This is followed by each pair sharing with the group what they experienced and learned, and they give each other feedback and receive feedback from the observers. Each pair goes through this process in turn.

CONCLUDING DISCUSSION

The facilitator leads the group discussion about the topic of the session and the learning process that they experienced – what they are taking away with them.

SECOND WORKSHOP –
DEVELOPING INTERPERSONAL COMMUNICATION SKILLS
Session 2 – Handling the Conversation
(For distribution to the group members)

HANDLING THE CONVERSATION

The conversation is a central tool in communication, in drawing closer to others and in building and deepening connections. The objective of the conversation – to create contact with another person, exchange information and ideas with him and make him feel that he matters to us.

EFFECTIVE HANDLING OF A CONVERSATION IS IMPORTANT BECAUSE IT:

- Encourages a friendly atmosphere around the connection.
- Enables accumulative experience in conversations, which lowers anxiety and strengthens our self-confidence.
- Increases the awareness of how we function in our ties with other people.

BASIC RULES FOR HANDLING A CONVERSATION:

- Do not interrupt the other person who is speaking, wait until he has finished (even if it is really hard!!).
- Maintain eye contact, to discern if your dialogue partner hasn't lost interest.
- Try to find a way of presenting the topic in a concentrated manner, without burdening the listener with too many small details.

- Use a language that is suitable to your dialogue partner.
- Use themes instead of topics, in order to raise interest. For example: "How can I convince my parents that I need more personal space and independence?" (theme), instead of: "Parent-child relationships" (topic).

THE TASK – PARTICIPATION IS MANDATORY

You are asked to initiate three conversations during the week, and write down in your journal a brief summary of their contents. Please write:

- What was easy for you and what was hard?
- What type of behavior helped draw your dialogue partner closer, and what type of behavior caused him to draw away?
- After the conversations have been recorded in the journals, the group meets to discuss what was written and to receive feedback.

The next stage: The group discusses a social or interpersonal theme. For example: Success in studies – Does it help, and in what way does it contribute toward integrating into society, both professionally and socially?

This is followed with giving feedback to the group members. It is important not to shy away from giving honest feedback, gently. (For example: Did one of the group members "hog" the discussion? Did a member remain silent and not contribute at all to the discussion? Did the group stick to the theme and the consensus? To what extent did they digress from it?, etc.). Also note what can be improved.

The session ends with light conversation over a cup of coffee.

SECOND WORKSHOP –
DEVELOPING INTERPERSONAL COMMUNICATION SKILLS
Session 3 – Handling a Conversation Leading to Bonding

INTRODUCTION

(Following a short discussion of the tasks from the previous session)

Understanding the basic principles of verbal communication is important to us all. First of all, we should take a moment to consider the circumstances of the conversation and understand its background data and significance. This includes the framework in which the conversation is taking place, the time framework and the degree of closeness or distance between the participants when their encounter begins. That is, what are the differences in the social status of the participants in the conversation (authority, friendship, closeness, formality or an open, coincidental conversation).

Data relating to the time allocated for talking and listening is important, as is the principle of "favoring" our dialogue partner, active listening, **avoiding an impulsive response** that **interrupts** our partner's words, etc. No less important are expressions of friendliness and bonding, such as: "It's great to see you"; "I enjoy your company, I've learned a lot of new things from you"; "I hope the feeling is mutual"; "I'd like to see you again soon"; "See you soon"; "Take care"; "Keep in touch"; "Thanks for everything," etc. The initial impression, when encountering a smiling conversational partner, impacts on the atmosphere of the conversation itself and the warm gestures of parting leave a meaningful memory of what has transpired. During the conversation, it is good to ask your partner if the topic under discussion interests him or perhaps he would prefer to change the subject. It is important to learn and practice certain issues, such as: How to join a conversation that is in process, meeting a new acquaintance, changing the subject politely (the facilitator encourages a short discussion on each of the above behaviorisms in order to help the participants internalize their significance).

EXPERIENCE A – ENGAGING IN CONVERSATION IN DIFFERENT SITUATIONS

The facilitator prepares cue cards with short vignettes describing encounters in different situations. Each card describes one encounter (these vignettes should be adapted to the group members). Here are some examples:

a. Two **high school students**, who haven't met before, meet at a club activity of some kind and start a conversation to get to know one another, which at the end of that day's activity will lead them to go out to have a drink together.

b. A **high school student** is invited by a girl from his class to study with her for an exam, they plan when and where they will study and ask about each other's study habits. They soon realize that their study habits are totally different, yet they want to develop their contact and examine ways for them to adjust to one another.

c. In a **high school** – A getting acquainted meeting between a student and his new homeroom teacher. The student wants to impress the teacher and the teacher wants to get to know the student and create a positive bond between them.

d. In a **high school** – A meeting between a student and a school counselor who doesn't know him. The student is very stressed and the counselor immediately senses this and encourages him to open up and tell her what it is that is bothering him. She is successful despite the fact that it is hard for him.

e. At the **university** – A chance meeting between two friends in the cafeteria, after not having seen each other for a long time, while both have experienced failures and successes in their studies, at work and social life.

f. In the **army** – As above, two soldiers, a boy and girl, meet by chance at the canteen and exchange their army experiences.

The group is divided into pairs. **After each exercise,** each pair discusses what took place and give each other feedback before the entire group. They then switch roles, and repeat the exercise. The facilitator will guide the exercise, and will observe and help solve problems as needed. The **concluding** discussion is the critical step of formulating and internalizing the individual learning process for each participant. This is done by having each group member in turn participate and express his feelings.

Note: In order to carry out all the exercises, this session requires more time. If time still remains, the facilitator can use it as he sees fit – opening a group discussion or additional exercises that fit the theme, etc.

SECOND WORKSHOP –
DEVELOPING INTERPERSONAL COMMUNICATION SKILLS

Session 3 – Handling a Conversation Leading to Creating Contact (For distribution to the group members)

WHAT ARE THE BASIC PRINCIPLES OF COMMUNICATION IN A CONVERSATION WHICH LEAD TO FORMING TIES?

- Understanding the relevance of the event – the conversation's framework conditions.
- Awareness of the time frame of the conversation.
- The degree of closeness or distance between the participants at the start of the encounter, evaluating the similarity or difference in their social status (authority, friendship, formal or friendly conversation).
- Skills in initiating a conversation:
  * Joining an ongoing conversation after clarifying its appropriateness.
  * Meeting a new acquaintance.
  * Changing the topic in a polite manner.
- The manner in which one handles himself during a conversation:
  * The time devoted to speaking and the time devoted to listening.
  * "Favoring" the dialogue partner and expressing friendship and bonding.
  * Refraining from an impulsive response that interrupts the partner's words.

* Active listening – check if the topic under discussion is of interest to the dialogue partner and if he is interested in continuing.

There is special significance to the beginning stage when accompanied by a pleasant smile, as well as to warm gestures when parting which form a meaningful memory ("I hope we see each other again," "We'll meet again soon," "When is it suitable for you?").

THE TASK – PARTICIPATION IS MANDATORY.

1. Choose three people with whom you will initiate a conversation – preferably people you are interested in having contact with. For example: a neighbor, a classmate, a colleague at work, a cousin, etc.

2. Write down a plan for each of these conversations:

- Introducing yourself and opening remarks ("I'm glad we met," etc.).
- Formulating the background of the conversation and what need it fulfills.
- The objective of the conversation.
- Phrasing the questions or requests.
- The preferred closure for the conversation, or what is expected to be gained at the conversation's end in regard to the connection formed.
- Words of parting.

3. At the group meeting, each person practices the role plays with another group member of his choice. In summing up, mutual feedback is given on how the exercise was implemented.

The session ends with light talk over a cup of coffee.

SECOND WORKSHOP –
DEVELOPING INTERPERSONAL COMMUNICATION SKILLS
Session 4 – Reciprocity and Cooperation

INTRODUCTION

We will begin with a short discussion on the process of fulfilling the tasks. We will then turn to the topic of this session – "Reciprocity and Cooperation" – with emphasis on the difficulties and benefits of reciprocity and cooperation.

The concept of 'reciprocity' includes three channels of giving and receiving:

Sharing ideas and being committed to achieving the shared goal.

Reciprocity in emotional communication – sharing feelings and emotions, via verbal and non-verbal gestures.

Giving and receiving at a constructive level, meaning: "I give you what I have that can be of help to you, and you give me what you have that can be of help to me." This principle applies to all levels of giving – from thinking and up to doing.

EXPERIENCE A

The major difficulties that disrupt communication, which basically serves to draw people closer and increase cooperation between them, stem from a number of reasons:

a. Difficulty in understanding and defining our own feelings and those of others.

b. A limited ability in understanding the thoughts, feelings and intentions of others.

c. A limited understanding of the **sophisticated nature** of reciprocal relationships in the adult world (white lies, half-truths, inability to defer gratification, generalizations, etc.).

d. A basic understanding only of non-verbal gestures and difficulty in deciphering the message they are communicating.

e. Not knowing or not understanding social codes.

f. Difficulty in internalizing the social rules that were learned and applying them in a flexible and appropriate manner to the context.

g. Focusing on details without addressing the wider picture (seeing the trees but not the forest).

h. Monopolizing the conversational space, without allowing room for others.

i. Difficulty in understanding the results or consequences of actions or behaviorisms of oneself or of others.

j. Mishaps in interpersonal communication resulting from an inability to open up and clarify misunderstandings.

The facilitator – Encourages the participants, following each item, to express their own perceptions and difficulties. He points out that these factors are learned throughout life and that one can always improve and become more proficient.

EXPERIENCE B – GIVING AND RECEIVING AS A MEANS OF DRAWING CLOSER

The facilitator describes a situation and the conversation that the participants engage in, exemplifying the process of trying to draw closer and cooperate, and its outcome.

Stage 1:

The facilitator: You notice that, during the breaks, one of your classmates sits alone in the corner of the cafeteria and drinks coffee, without relating to his surroundings. What do you learn about him from this behavior? This is a student whom you like. What will you say to him when you approach his table? Write in your notebooks two possible conversation openers.

After reading the group members' suggestions, the facilitator presents other possibilities, such as: "May I join you?," "Would you like me to bring you something to go with the coffee?" (a careful, tactful approach that also demonstrates empathy).

In the event that you are not invited to join him: "I understand you wish to be alone. That's fine with me, it happens to me too, but don't hesitate to turn to me when you can."

To the facilitator: During the group discussion, you can help those members whose suggested responses were inappropriate, by demonstrating a better option.

Stage 2:

The following day, in the cafeteria, that same student asks you to join him. He explains that he was in a bad mood the day before, because on his way to work someone had pushed himself into line before him, which caused him to be late and be reprimanded. All this occurred because the bus door had closed shut before he could get on the bus.

The facilitator: 'How would you react to this situation? Write down two suggestions, one useful and one not useful'. Emphasize that the non-useful response increases one's frustration, as it is misunderstood. The group members should be asked to relate an incident that angered or saddened them and how they would want others to react. Then a **concluding discussion** should be held that relates to the different methods that are helpful.

SECOND WORKSHOP –
DEVELOPING INTERPERSONAL COMMUNICATION SKILLS
Session 4 – Reciprocity and Cooperation
(For distribution to the group members)

THE CONCEPT OF 'RECIPROCITY' INCLUDES A NUMBER OF CHANNELS OF GIVING AND RECEIVING:

1. **Sharing ideas** and being committed to achieving the shared goal.
2. **Reciprocity in emotional communication** – sharing feelings and emotions, via verbal and non-verbal gestures.
3. **Giving and receiving** in a manner that is helpful to both sides.

Reasons for the difficulties that disrupt communication, which is meant to draw people closer and increase their cooperation:

1. Difficulty in understanding and defining our own feelings and those of others.
2. A limited ability in understanding the thoughts, feelings and intentions of others.
3. A limited understanding of the **sophisticated nature** of reciprocal relationships in the adult world (white lies, half-truths, inability to defer gratification, generalizations, etc.).
4. A basic understanding only of non-verbal gestures and difficulty in deciphering their communication message.
5. Not knowing or not understanding social codes.
6. Difficulty in internalizing the social rules that were learned

and to apply them in a flexible and appropriate manner to the context.

7. Focusing on details without including them in the wider picture (seeing the trees but not the forest).

8. Monopolizing the conversational space, without allowing room for others.

9. Difficulty in understanding the results and consequences of actions or behaviorisms of oneself or of others.

10. Difficulty in opening up and clarifying misunderstandings through mutual effort.

THE TASK – PARTICIPATION IS MANDATORY

At the group meeting, each person in turn relates to the others an incident that made him angry, sad, hurt, etc. The members listen and try to react in a way that will help him overcome. For example: By relating a similar incident and how it made them feel, and how others would feel or react if it had happened to them. Support is empowering and this is an opportunity to experience it. It is important not to skim over differences of opinion, but rather discuss them in depth and matter-of-factly.

This is followed by light conversation over a cup of coffee.

SECOND WORKSHOP –
DEVELOPING INTERPERSONAL COMMUNICATION SKILLS

Session 5– Confrontations: How To Resolve Them and
Develop Tolerance Toward Others

"In that place where we are in the right,
no spring flowers will grow."
Yehuda Amichai

INTRODUCTION

(Following a short discussion of the tasks)

Confrontations are situations that grow out of disagreement, opposition, frustration and anger. We are usually wary of confrontations in order to avoid being hurt, to avoid aggression and destructiveness and also out of a natural fear that things may get out of hand. Nonetheless, confrontation is a natural process in interpersonal relationships. Expressing feelings, ideas, opinions, intentions, goals and plans is the basic way of giving expression to one's self. Therefore, in every interpersonal encounter there is a chance of disagreement between the parties involved. Each of us accumulates experience in coping with confrontation and can acquire tools based on interpersonal communication skills. As mentioned, confrontations are a natural phenomenon in relationships between people. Only he who lives on a desert island or remains secluded in his home is never called upon to confront such situations. Therefore, social skills that impact upon solving conflicts are essential for us all.

EXPERIENCE A – A DISCUSSION ABOUT EFFECTIVE COPING WITH CONFLICT (VIA THE FOLLOWING ITEMS):

1. Conflict is a natural phenomenon, and in order to learn to deal with it, it has to be experienced, not avoided.

2. Our basic assumption here is that the group members agree that it is okay to disagree.

3. Conflicts are hard to resolve, if the energies of those involved are targeted at one thing – to win the argument and be proven right.

4. During the process of confrontation, when the discussion is clean from competitiveness, a better understanding is created between one side and the other (see item 2).

5. With active listening it is easier to better understand our dialogue partner in an argument: What is it that he wants, what does he feel and what does he need? (see item 4).

6. Such an understanding, especially if it is mutual, facilitates negotiation and changing positions and perceptions, toward consolidating principles and ways of cooperation (see items 4,5).

EXERCISES:

The facilitator asks of the group members to recall an event of significant confrontation, including the feelings and emotions it first aroused, then think of its progression and how it ended. The facilitator reads to the group each of the following questions and some possible answers, and instructs the group members to write them down in their notebooks **and rank them.**

1. **What frightened me in the confrontation event? The following are examples of some possible answers:** I will lose the argument and end up feeling embarrassed; The argument will become heated and I will have to absorb insults; I won't know how to get out of it honorably; The argument will get completely out of hand; I will lose control; I will be exposed; I will be rejected; I will show weakness; and other such similar answers.

2. **What challenges me in a conflict situation? The following are examples of some possible answers:** There is a high energy level in the room; this is my chance to show who I am; it's better to be involved in an interaction of disagreement than to have no contact with others; it's a chance to blow off steam; and other feelings.

3. **What do you feel when the conflict has been resolved? The following are examples of some possible answers:** Exhaustion, satisfaction, a sense of gratification for the understanding I was granted, a sense of widening my horizons in understanding the other, high motivation for cooperation, drawing closer rather than distancing, an opportunity to start on a new path, etc.

The facilitator then invites the participants to talk about each of the above topics, in the above order of the questions. He encourages the others to respond and tell about their own experiences. The facilitator will navigate the discussion, and help those who are having difficulty to formulate their responses and feelings, and finally he will contribute his own perceptions.

EXPERIENCE B – FROM THAT PLACE WHERE WE ARE IN THE RIGHT, NOTHING GOOD WILL GROW: EXERCISES IN CONFLICT SITUATIONS

The facilitator prepares a number of themes that can be debated, adjusted to the age and education of the group members. **For example:** "Should all the religious and ultra-Orthodox young men be obligated, without exception, to serve in the army?" He presents the topic to the entire group and asks who is pro and who is con, then chooses the respondents accordingly.

1. The facilitator chooses a pair from the group to debate the theme and appoints the person to argue "pro" and the one to argue "con." He guides each of them separately and secretly, that **in no case** are they to reach agreement with one another. The debate is carried out in front of the group members as observers. Once the debate has reached its end or is ended by the facilitator, a discussion is held regarding what the debaters experienced, and the observers express their opinions and what they felt.

2. The facilitator prepares another theme for another pair. For example: "Do you think we should retreat from the Golan Heights and remove settlements in return for peace?" Here too he prompts each one of the pair, pro or con, instructing them to insist on their views, yet to also try and find out from the other, "Why do you think that?," or "Explain to me what you mean" or "How would you feel if you were in that place?," thus creating a greater understanding of the other's opinion. The exercise doesn't necessarily end in agreement or by fully identifying with the opposing argument, but rather with phrases such as: "There's something in what you're saying," "I have to think about it," "It would be good to check what

others think and what their arguments are." That is, the argument ends with an openness and growing closeness to one another's position. The pair and the observers will share their opinions and feelings with the group.

3. The facilitator prepares another theme, which contains an element of uncertainty: "To what extent should the government be obligated to help the country's weaker populations, and what is the responsibility of the families and the social volunteer organizations in the community?". The facilitator instructs the pair chosen to debate this issue, to express their positions and reach **a joint formula** that will satisfy both sides. A discussion then follows on the formula that was reached as the observers express their feelings.

CONCLUSION

What are the differences between the three confrontations, in terms of the outcome, the consequences and feelings? What have we learned from the exercises on conflict in general, and about ourselves in particular?

SECOND WORKSHOP –
DEVELOPING INTERPERSONAL COMMUNICATION SKILLS

Session 5– Confrontations: How To Resolve Them
and Develop Tolerance Toward Others
(For distribution to the group members)

WHAT ARE CONFRONTATIONS?

- Confrontations are situations that grow out of disagreement, opposition, frustration and anger.
- We are usually wary of confrontations, to avoid being hurt, to avoid aggression.
- Confrontations are a natural process of disagreements, conflict of interests and conflicting perceptions in interpersonal relationships - expressing feelings, ideas and opinions is the basic way of giving expression to one's self, even when there is disagreement. The manner in which a confrontation is handled is more important than its contents.
- One can acquire tools for managing conflicts, based on interpersonal communication skills.

IMPORTANT POINTS FOR EFFECTIVE HANDLING OF CONFLICTS

1. Conflict is a natural phenomenon, and in order to learn from it, it has to be experienced, and not avoided.
2. The basic assumption is that the group members agree that it is okay to disagree.
3. A conflict becomes difficult to resolve when those involved want to win the argument and be proven right.

4. When the confrontation is void of competitiveness, a better understanding is created between one side and the other.

5. Active listening helps to better understand our dialogue partner in an argument.

6. Mutual acceptance facilitates negotiation, and changing positions and perceptions toward consolidating principles and ways of cooperation.

THE TASK – PARTICIPATION IS MANDATORY

Write in your notebooks about events in which you were involved in a conflict:

- What took place?
- How did the confrontation begin?
- What did you feel during the confrontation?
- Discuss this in the group session.
- Remember – there is no one correct formula: Different people can experience the same event in different ways.

The session ends with light conversation over a cup of coffee.

SECOND WORKSHOP –
DEVELOPING INTERPERSONAL COMMUNICATION SKILLS
Session 6 – The Effective Management of Anger

INTRODUCTION

Anger is a feeling that grows from both internal and external factors. It rises from an external stimulus that is caused sometimes by a specific event or another person, and at times it is an internal stimulus that arises within us. Anger is like "a stray bullet looking for a target," that is, aimed at a specific situation or person. The object of the anger can be the person himself who feels angry, when he has unresolved internal conflicts. Anger is a feeling that usually grows out of frustration, when things didn't work out as desired, expected or planned.

If the frustrated person can find a way of calming himself down at this early stage, and examine what it is that is frustrating him and why, he will be able to put things into proportion and handle the problem without outbursts of anger. The alternative is an immediate release of unpleasant energy. This energy may create a reaction that has an aggressive base to it (from yelling, swearing and cursing to actual physical harm to property or another person). All of us have experienced the nature of frustration since childhood, in the social sphere as well, and we are sensitive to interpersonal situations of tension. When coping with difficulties in deciphering the social map, the level of frustration is high and, as a result, what may unfold is perceived at times as a personal insult, even though that isn't the case. The energies from anger are overwhelming and create ineffective responses that achieve the opposite effect of what the angry person wished to gain. When there is no regulation or control of one's anger, two prominent reactions ensue:

The first is a reaction of escape in its different forms, i.e., denial, repression, disconnecting from the situation, etc. Turning one's anger inwardly (self-restraint) may have undesirable effects on the emotional well-being of the angry person.

The second is channeling the anger toward others. Frustrations resulting from a lack of understanding or acceptance from one's environment give rise to anger and bitterness, leaving us overwhelmed and exhausted. An immediate and direct clarification of one's anger can provide the angry person with immediate relief. In contrast, demonstrating anger (raising one's voice, threatening, etc.) is usually perceived as threatening and causes distancing between the discussants.

The desired response should be expressed by the angry party informing his dialogue partner, in a calm manner, how he feels. This is an effective way of achieving one's goal without locking up one's anger inside. The following experiences are designed to provide tools for coping effectively with situations of anger.

STEPS FOR THE EFFECTIVE MANAGEMENT OF ANGER

The effective examination and processing of anger should be done in three stages:

a. Identifying and finding **the circumstance or stimulus** that incited anger: Is it something that happens to you repeatedly, such as when: Making a mistake, losing something, not getting what you wanted, waiting a long time for something, etc. Perhaps the stimulus is internal, such as: A lack of sleep, hunger, physical pain, failure, etc. Other stimuli that may cause anger should be found and identified, such as various behaviorisms, laws, norms, injustice, unfairness, etc.

a. **Identifying thoughts** – How you perceive or understand what has happened. For example: Was it a general expression of opinion or a desire to hurt you personally? (in which case your anger will increase). Try to get help from a friend or family member to review how you tend to interpret similar events.

a. **Identifying feelings** – Are you angry, sad, scared, insulted, hurt, frustrated, disappointed in yourself?

Identifying the anger-triggering stimuli will enable a change in your manner of thinking about anger and how you handle it, and help you find ways to calm down when angry and learning to talk about it instead of letting loose without control. **Try to change** the level of stimulus, through your own initiative. For example, if you have been given a task at work that is beyond your skills, **ask for help** instead of turning your anger toward your supervisor. It is important to find effective ways to help you calm down when you are unable to avoid feeling angry. Since the ability to think logically is temporarily suspended by your anger, it is recommended that in those moments you focus your attention on a relaxing activity and engage in an internal dialogue with the anger, to balance it out and place things into proper proportion.

EXPERIENCE A – IDENTIFYING ANGER-TRIGGERING STIMULI

a. The group begins a discussion on the personal and interpersonal significance of acquiring control over one's anger.

b. Each participant does his own brainstorming, in which he

writes in his notebook situations and behaviorisms that angered him. These should include a short description of the situation and **identifying** the stimulus in each event that angered him, as well as what he thought and how others reacted.

c. Upon completing the above activity, the facilitator reads aloud the following stimuli, listed below, and asks the group members if these include additional anger-triggering situations that are familiar to them. Each member adds to his list those stimuli that he identifies with himself.

EXTERNAL STIMULI	INTERNAL STIMULI
Overload at work	Insomnia
Being criticized	Frustrations from myself
When I've "been had"	Self-criticism
Passing from an interesting activity to one Less interesting	Memories from the past
Losing at a game	Sensory stimuli
When I don't get what I want	Hunger

EXPERIENCE B – STRATEGIES FOR SELF-CALMING

The facilitator suggests to the participants the following strategies:

1. Internal dialogue – Think of mantras that will remind you to relax, such as: "I don't want to ruin something that I will want later on"; "It isn't worth it," etc.

2. Remove yourself from the situation – Count to ten, take deep breaths, imagine pleasant things, talk to a friend, write, listen to music, etc. it is recommended to practice this repeatedly over time, and adapt yourself to both public and private situations.

3. You've calmed down? Try to think of an appropriate way to correct the mistakes you made when you were angry (Reconcile? Apologize? Explain? Etc.).

EXPERIENCE C – THE PREFERRED ALTERNATIVE: TALK ABOUT YOUR ANGER INSTEAD OF IMMEDIATELY RELEASING EMOTIONS

The group is divided into pairs. The person in the role of the angry partner is talking with his older brother, who didn't want to take him along when he went with his friends to the movies. After he has calmed himself down, the angry partner sets up a time for them to meet and discuss what happened, without being under pressure. He explains that he wants to talk to him **in private**. He should talk **about himself** calmly: "What do I feel, what happened during the event, and why I feel the way I do." After that, he is to listen to his dialogue partner **without interrupting**, and only after the latter has finished, the angry dialogue initiator responds once again, until both have fully made their points and reached a mutual understanding.

CONCLUSION

What have I learned about myself and about managing and channeling my anger? How can angry energies be channeled toward positive action, thus experiencing self-empowerment? What suits me best?

All the group members speak in turn, so that everyone has a chance to express himself. The facilitator adds his own explanations and perceptions.

SECOND WORKSHOP –
DEVELOPING INTERPERSONAL COMMUNICATION SKILLS
Session 6 – The Effective Management of Anger
(For distribution to the group members)

INTRODUCTION
- Anger is triggered by both internal and external factors.
- Anger is targeted at either a person or a specific situation.
- Anger derives usually from frustration, when things don't happen as we wished, expected or planned.
- When coping with difficulties in deciphering the social map, at times what takes place is interpreted as a personal insult, which then leads to anger, frustration and hurt feelings.

DEALING WITH ANGER
- We usually release our anger outwardly aggressively (yelling, cursing, etc.), or channel inwardly toward ourselves the unpleasant or painful energies (self-criticism, feelings of guilt, etc.).
- The alternative: Calm ourselves down, examine what causes our frustration and why.
- Thus we will be able to place things back into proportion and deal with the problems without angry outbursts.

WHERE THERE IS A LACK OF REGULATION OR CONTROL OF ONE'S ANGER, SEVERAL MANIFEST REACTIONS ENSUE:
- An escape response – denial, repression, disconnection, etc.

- Internalizing anger may bring on depression.
- Channeling our anger toward others – frustrations result from a lack of understanding and acceptance by our environment, causing anger and bitterness, and leaving us overwhelmed and exhausted.
- An immediate release of the anger will relieve us, but may leave in its wake long-term interpersonal damage – demonstrating anger is perceived as threatening and therefore creates a distancing between those engaged in a dialogue.

STEPS FOR THE EFFECTIVE MANAGEMENT OF ANGER:

An effective examination and processing of anger are implemented in three stages:

1. Identifying and finding **the circumstance or stimulus** that triggered the anger: Is it something that happens to you repeatedly? Is it an internal or external stimulus?
2. **Identifying thoughts** – How you perceive or understand what has happened. Try to get help from a friend or family member to review how you tend to interpret similar events.
3. **Identifying feelings** – Are you angry, or perhaps is it another emotion that you are experiencing?

STRATEGIES FOR SELF CALMING:

1. Identifying anger-triggering stimuli will facilitate a change in the level of the stimulus. For example: If you were given a task at work that is beyond your capabilities, **ask for help** instead of getting angry at your supervisor.
2. Internal dialogue – Think of mantras that will help you relax ("It isn't worth it," etc.).
3. Remove yourself from the situation – Count to ten, take deep

breaths, imagine pleasant things, write, listen to music, etc. it is recommended to practice this repeatedly over time.

THE TASK – PARTICIPATION IS MANDATORY

Write in your notebook about three situations in which you became angry.

How did you behave, and how did the source of your anger - a person or your surroundings - react?

How could you have solved the situation in a different way?

Discuss these events at the group session and together suggest the correct way for handling anger.

The session ends with light conversation over a cup of coffee.

SECOND WORKSHOP –
DEVELOPING INTERPERSONAL COMMUNICATION SKILLS
Session 7 – Self-Advocacy

INTRODUCTION

The theme we will be addressing today is that of **self-advocacy:** What is it and how do we apply it? Self-advocacy is a tool that we use in order to present ourselves to others effectively, without being apologetic or defensive.

The basic conditions that are mandatory for self-advocacy are: Reasonable **self–awareness** and the advocator's acceptance of **himself**. It is important that he have a reasonable understanding of the **context** of the event in which he advocates himself.

SELF-AWARENESS, SELF-ACCEPTANCE AND UNDERSTANDING THE CONTEXT

No person can advocate for himself without self-awareness. This awareness is the outcome of a relatively **consolidated self-identity.** It is a situation in which the advocator has a clear picture of "Who I am and what I am." This includes a recognition of his talents, as well as his ability to find and define those areas in which he has difficulty in coping alone.

EXPERIENCE A

At this stage, the facilitator asks the participants to open their journals and write down:

a. Skills, talents, successes and supporting circumstances
b. Coping with my difficulties and effective solutions.
c. Traits that I value in myself.

Advocacy can be done by the individual himself either via talking or writing, or by someone else who assists him. There are situations in which the need for self-advocacy arises in the course of a conversation with someone else, at which point it should be implemented spontaneously. This is not an easy situation, but for someone with self-awareness it is easier to express his talents, advantages, accomplishments and successes – all of which help in achieving the goal.

When self-advocacy is planned in advance, one can present the material either orally or in writing (and also be helped by people who are well acquainted with the advocator). Writing things out allows us to use this text in future encounters as well. It is highly important to have a reasonable understanding of the context in which the advocacy talk will evolve. For example: For those who are seeking employment, clearly it is fitting and desirable to research and learn everything possible about the organization or company to which the candidate has been called for a job interview. The advocator should have all the necessary data about the workplace in order to present himself in a manner most suited to the organization that will be interviewing him. We wish to stress that a clear definition of the objective of one's self-advocacy should fit the understanding of the goals, intentions, preferences and needs of the other side. Here is another example: When getting acquainted with **a new friend**, the chances of this developing into a long-term friendship or even a couple relationship are far better, after a successful self-advocacy. Here too, it is preferable to obtain preliminary data about the person you are about to meet and adapt your advocacy or self presentation to the nature and purpose of the meeting. In the above example, it is a meeting for making a personal acquaintance and therefore the style will be that of an informal discussion between equals, with an honest self presentation and with demonstrations of **interest in the other person**.

EXPERIENCE B – WEAK SPOTS

The group members are divided into threes, to examine in retrospect situations in which they tried to self-advocate: Did they avoid self presentation or fail in their self presentation in one way or another? Were they stressed, anxious, confused or lose control? The facilitator talks in turn with each of the groups and helps them address the difficulties that have arisen. Discussion should also include partial or complete successes and if these occurred in a formal interview or a friendly meeting.

In the forum, each group of three reports one of the difficulties discussed, in order to receive additional feedback.

The facilitator concludes what has taken place in the process of this experience and what can be learned from it.

EXPERIENCE C – ROLE-PLAY

Four volunteers for role-play will be divided into two pairs. Each pair will prepare a job interview or an interview for college entrance. Each pair will present its assignment to the group, wherein one is the interviewee (the advocator), the other is the interviewer (the authority). They will then demonstrate the same situation again, switching roles. When they have finished, they will share their experience with the group, and the group will respond with comments, disagreements and feedback.

To the facilitator: This session is of notable importance toward the participants' success in their **careers,** in social contacts and in general. Therefore, it is **recommended** to add another **thirty minutes** to the time frame, as pre-arranged with the group.

SECOND WORKSHOP –
DEVELOPING INTERPERSONAL COMMUNICATION SKILLS
Session 7 – Self-Advocacy
(For distribution to the group members)

WHAT IS SELF-ADVOCACY?

Self-advocacy is a tool that we use to present ourselves to others effectively, without being apologetic or defensive.

EXAMPLES OF SITUATIONS IN WHICH WE ARE CALLED UPON FOR SELF-ADVOCACY:

- **Planned situations:** Presenting ourselves to someone whom we want to accept us (a job interview, a new acquaintance). For such situations we can prepare our self-advocacy in advance, either orally or in writing, and enlist help from people close to us.
- **Spontaneous situations:** An unplanned encounter with someone, during which we are called upon to advocate for ourselves.

CONDITIONS FOR SUCCESSFUL SELF-ADVOCACY:

- Self-awareness is important in presenting ourselves success-fully – toward that purpose, a person must know who he is and what he is, that is, to recognize his talents and abilities, yet to also identify those areas in which he has difficulty in coping alone.
- Understanding the context: For example, for a job interview,

we should gather as much data as we can about the organization we want to be hired by.

- Awareness of others: To present ourselves successfully, we have to understand what it is that the listener wants, so that we can suit our self presentation to meet his interests. For example, at a job interview, we will present those traits of ours that fit the organization's needs. Another example: Getting socially acquainted. Here too it is best to know as much as possible about the new person we are meeting. It will be a conversation between equals, and we will emphasize an honest presentation of ourselves and demonstrate interest in others.

THE TASK – PARTICIPATION IS MANDATORY

The group meets to practice self-advocacy before an authoritative figure. Each group member will suggest an authoritative figure. Some suggestions: A scene in which the authority figure is a supervisor at work; a school principal vs. a student; a school principal vs. a teacher; a team leader at work; a job interview, etc. The school principal or work supervisor may be tough and firm, whereas another is curious and nosy, a third is all smiles and polite, a fourth is accepting and encouraging. After the roles are determined, the group is divided into pairs, one role-playing the interviewee and one the interviewer (the authority figure). Each interviewee tries to focus on the tactics of self-advocacy and cope with the challenges he faces from the authority figure.

1. School principal vs. teacher: An evaluation meeting of the teacher's work during the past year.
2. Work supervisor vs. employee: An interview to evaluate

whether the employee is suited for promotion in his work.

3. Getting acquainted with a potential friend or mate.

4. Team leader vs. employee: Checking if the employee can serve as the team leader, replacing the current leader who is leaving.

The group members help each pair after their presentation with feedback or alternative suggestions. Each person plays both the role of authority and the role of self-advocacy.

The session ends with light conversation over a cup of coffee.

SECOND WORKSHOP –
DEVELOPING INTERPERSONAL COMMUNICATION SKILLS
Session 8 – Effective Feedback

INTRODUCTION

We will begin with a brief discussion of the tasks from the previous session. Today we will first discuss and clarify what feedback is and present it as an effective tool in interpersonal communication. Following that, the participants will practice giving feedback.

FEEDBACK

Feedback is interpersonal information that one discussant shares with another. The one giving the feedback relates to what his dialogue partner has said and how he behaved, and shares with him his thoughts and criticisms. Feedback is a two-way communication mechanism between an individual and a group or between an individual and his dialogue partner.

EFFECTIVE FEEDBACK

Feedback is a very significant way of enabling us to learn how we are perceived by others and expand our own self-awareness, and through this to strive for change. It helps us consolidate an understanding of our abilities and strengths and serves as a mirror of sorts that helps us identify where we were mistaken and what we should change or improve.

CONDITIONS FOR IMPLEMENTING FEEDBACK:

1. The person giving the feedback considers what is the most suitable time and context for transmitting the information.

2. The discussion and the relationship are ripe for giving feedback at a given point in time.

3. The person giving feedback recognizes what the abilities of the recipient are, and **opens** the discussion by first expressing support and positive reinforcements of those traits, such as: "It was easy for me to identify with what you said when…" or "I really enjoy your humor," etc. This style creates a positive and open atmosphere for accepting feedback that suggests change.

4. The recipient is attentive and open to what the giver has to say, and the situation facilitates mutuality in their relationship.

5. The person giving feedback marks his retreat when the receiver shows signs of not being capable of listening or internalizing what is being said ("I don't feel like talking about it," etc.).

6. Effective feedback calls for courage, openness, frankness and empathy from both sides.

THE ADDED VALUE OF EFFECTIVE FEEDBACK

1. It is an effective tool for cooperation, clarification and deepening of relationships.

2. It helps maintain flowing and open relationships of give-and-take, and promotes closeness between the dialogue partners.

3. It serves as an efficient solution for misunderstandings and conflicts in both temporary and ongoing relationships.

A STYLE THAT FACILITATES AND PROMOTES EFFECTIVENESS

1. Every feedback **begins** with a statement that is phrased in the singular pronoun, "I." Examples: "I have the impression that..."; "I feel that..."; "I assume that..."; "If I'm not mistaken, there is another option..." Remember that every statement which begins with the singular pronoun 'you' is often perceived at the very start of the sentence as accusatory, which in turn creates **antagonism** and disrupts the receiver's ability to absorb and digest the feedback that is meant to help him.

2. In order to avoid such obstacles, it is important that every feedback ends with a question: "What do you think?" or "What would you say about that?" or "How do you feel about what I said?" or "Would you like us to continue to clarify this together?" This inviting style of expression opens up the dialogue and broadcasts an empathic and respectful approach.

EXPERIENCE A

Each group member writes down on a sheet of paper a short message as feedback to one of the other group members and hands it to him. The message will be called "Snacks for the Way." Its contents will include a reflection that will help the recipient learn about himself. The feedback will be phrased in a personal tone to the recipient.

An important reminder: **Before** any feedback that hints at a need for improvement, there should first be **an introduction** that lays out **the capabilities** of the recipient. This will help increase his readiness to listen and accept what will follow. For example: "I very much appreciate your ability to listen. And I'm **learning from you** how not to interrupt the other person who is speaking. However, I suggest that you moderate your style of speaking which at times is harsh and may…"

EXPERIENCE B

An exercise in feedback, done in pairs. Whoever has received written feedback will initiate a dialogue with the one who gave it to him. As a pair, they will refer to what was written and discuss it. The recipient of the feedback will respond to what his partner has said and a discussion will follow until the matter is concluded. Following that, the observers will react and add their own evaluation. The facilitator will see to it that each group member is linked to another member and that everyone participates.

CONCLUDING DISCUSSION

Each pair reports to the group about their experience: How did it go? Was it hard? How did they cope? What did they learn about feedback in general, and about themselves in particular? The facilitator guides the discussion and ends with **feedback for the group** of what he has observed and shares his conclusions with them.

SECOND WORKSHOP –
DEVELOPING INTERPERSONAL COMMUNICATION SKILLS
Session 8 – Effective Feedback
(For distribution to the group members)

a. Feedback is a two-way communication mechanism between an individual and a group or between an individual and his dialogue partner.

b. Feedback helps us learn how we are perceived by others, and helps us consolidate perceptions about ourselves and identify our mistakes and what we should strive to change.

c. For effective feedback, there is need for courage, openness, frankness and empathy from both sides.

d. The person giving feedback considers what is the most suitable timing and context for transmitting the information

e. Feedback maintains open relationships, mutuality and closeness between the dialogue partners, and facilitates resolving both temporary and ongoing misunderstandings and conflicts.

f. The person giving feedback always begins by indicating and reinforcing the recipient's abilities, thus creating an atmosphere which lets him be open and attentive to recommended changes.

g. Every feedback begins with a statement that is phrased in the singular pronoun, "I." Examples: "**I** have the impression that…"; "**I** feel that…"; "**I** assume that…"; "If **I'm** not mistaken, there is another option…"

h.   A statement that begins with the singular pronoun 'you' is perceived as accusatory, which creates **antagonism** and hinders the effectiveness of the feedback.

i.   It is important to end with a request for the recipient's reaction: "What do you think?" or "How do you feel about what I said?" or "Would you like us to continue to clarify this together?" Such an ending emphasizes empathy and respect and invites continued discussion.

THE TASK – PARTICIPATION IS MANDATORY

The group meets in a quiet, comfortable venue. Each member prepares at home a written feedback for each of the members of the group. The text is phrased according to the general guidelines and precautions discussed with the facilitator at the session. The feedback will be presented before the group, therefore its content and style must be suited to the sensitivity of the recipient.

The meeting ends with light conversation over a cup of coffee.

SECOND WORKSHOP –
DEVELOPING INTERPERSONAL COMMUNICATION SKILLS
Session 9 – Deciphering Emotions, Intentions and Thoughts in Relationships
(Via a viewing of the Coen brothers' film, A Serious Man)

INTRODUCTION

During the next two sessions, the learning process will be based on the group members' joint viewing of the indicated film, as this film's plot is intertwined with a variegated gallery of relationships between the different characters. Additionally, it reflects interpersonal situations in a variety of contexts – couples, parents and children, authority figures in the school and the community, neighbors, etc. The facilitator will pause the showing of the film every once in a while and encourage a group discussion of the film's characters, their relationships with their families, their neighbors, friends, etc. In addition, the facilitator will call attention to the language beyond the words, with a discussion of the facial expressions and/or body language in a given frame.

RULES FOR VIEWING THE FILM AND ENSUING DISCUSSION

1. The basic assumption is that there are no unequivocal answers.
2. The different interpretations contribute to reviewing and analyzing what is taking place in the minds of the main characters and in their relationships.
3. Each group member listens to the other members' impres-

sions with maximum openness.

4. All the data that can be gathered from an analyzed event should be considered: The context, the relationships, the cultural, familial, economic, communal and social background.

5. A careful study should be made of the facial expressions and the eyes, the positions and movements of the body limbs, as well as the "behavioral language" (supportive, threatening, etc.).

6. All the cues should be deciphered interactively, in order to obtain the most intelligent understanding about each character, the relationships between the characters and their subsequent outcome.

7. A discussion is held on the emotions, thoughts and intentions of the main characters and their impact on the interpersonal relationships.

THE TASK – PARTICIPATION IS MANDATORY

The group agrees upon an appropriate venue for a picnic and organizes itself accordingly. The facilitator helps out as needed.

SECOND WORKSHOP –
DEVELOPING INTERPERSONAL COMMUNICATION SKILLS

Session 10 - Deciphering Emotions, Intentions and
Thoughts in Relationships (Continued)

INTRODUCTION

This session begins with a short summing up of what was learned in the first part, we will then continue with a viewing of the second part of the film, *A Serious Man*.

The film raises questions and conjectures regarding the nature of the relationships between the film's main characters. The discussion focuses on how honest or fake the relationships are, on the arrogance, etc.

The **discussion** emphasizes the empathy reflected in the plot and the various ways of using our **empathy** in order to understand what the other person is experiencing. The facilitator encourages the group members to utilize all the cues at their disposal from the non-verbal behavior of the characters in the film (context, physical clues, etc.) and translate them into an empathic understanding of the nature of his or her feelings and intentions at a given moment.

From a didactic standpoint, half the time of this session is devoted to watching the film, with pauses for analyzing situations, a general discussion of the film, its relevance and additional perceptions. Internalizing what has been understood from viewing the film is done via a cognitive processing of the experience, as a group discussion. The facilitator guides the discussion and presents his own perceptions and conclusions.

The second half of the session is devoted to a concluding discussion – at this stage, the facilitator asks each member in turn to express how he feels in the group, what he has learned about himself, what has the comradery in the group contributed, what he would like to add or change, etc.

It should be noted that this is an opportunity for the facilitator to learn from the group members.

It is recommended that the facilitator first encourage volunteers among the members to express themselves, and after that, to invite the other members to talk. it is extremely important that everyone expresses himself at this concluding discussion.

SECOND WORKSHOP –
DEVELOPING INTERPERSONAL COMMUNICATION SKILLS
SESSION 10 – Deciphering Emotions, Intentions and Thoughts in Relationships (Continued)
(For distribution to the group members)

THE TASK

The group members meet for a shared entertainment event of their choosing. Participation is **mandatory** – as usual. The facilitator informs the members of the exact details of the event. In nice weather, it is recommended to have a picnic somewhere pleasant (a park, on the beach).

The organizers see to the planning of the event and inform everyone of the details.

Have a Great Time!

SESSION 11 - COMPLETING EXERCISES & BRINGING OPEN ISSUES TO CLOSURE

SESSION 12 – CONCLUSION & INTEGRATION OF THE MATERIALS LEARNED

WORKSHOPS FOR DEVELOPING SOCIAL LIFE SKILLS FOR ADULTS WITH ASPERGER'S (ASD)

THIRD WORKSHOP – DEVELOPING SOCIAL LIFE SKILLS

We are all different from each other, but all equal to one another

INTRODUCTION

Social skills derive from the internalization and application of behavior codes in human relationships. These include a variety of culturally-linked interpersonal gestures, as well as accepted general gestures in the different cultures. Included are also the accepted codes of behavior for first or chance encounters with new people or old acquaintances, in private meetings or at larger gatherings. Internalizing these codes constitutes the basis of neurotypical behavior and upgrades the abilities of each one of us to integrate into society and foster friendships.

Adults with Asperger's (ASD) usually have difficulty in comprehending and applying the social codes. This difficulty is at the root of their social problems. They often initiate contact or respond in an inappropriate and even hurtful manner, where all they actually wanted and intended was just to connect with the other person, and perhaps also send a reminder: "I too am here" or "I also have something to contribute to this conversation." Unfortunately, the neurotypical society does not understand the source of their mistakes and responds by ignoring the speaker or being critical and at times even by excluding them. In this situation one misunderstanding leads to another and the adult with

Asperger's (ASD) is left in a state of uncertainty, which may develop into anxiety and depression. Simply put, he cannot identify what it is that he did wrong and for what he is being punished.

The objective of this workshop is to help the group members understand the source of this endless cycle of repeated mistakes in neurotypical behavior, the uncertainty they create and the anxiety and depression that follow. The frequently adopted and undesirable solution is found in their withdrawal and avoidance of social contacts as a survival mechanism.

THIRD WORKSHOP – DEVELOPING SOCIAL LIFE SKILLS

Session 1 – Awareness of Social Codes in Everyday Life

INTRODUCTION

Social behaviorisms are naturally based upon social norms. They do not come in written form as regulations, but rather are acquired through the experience of daily life. A deviation from these norms may disrupt the process of communication and contact. That is why it is necessary and important to become familiar with the social codes.

In this session, we will practice social situations, with emphasis on the codes of neurotypical interpersonal behavior.

EXPERIENCE A – SOCIAL CODES IN EVERYDAY LIFE
(PRELIMINARY DISCUSSION)

The facilitator distributes to the participants a list of the social codes. The group is divided into pairs. Each pair reviews the list and marks with a plus sign (+) the codes they are familiar with and understand. The other codes are to be marked with a minus sign (-), for whatever reason: The code is difficult, complicated, embarrassing, unclear, unacceptable to me, etc. Each pair discusses those codes marked with a minus sign. Each code they have been unable to decipher is brought before the group forum, in the last part of the exercise.

EXPERIENCE B – MEETING WITH FRIENDS

Two friends from the far past who haven't met in a very long time meet at a café. **The task** for both is to create a pleasant conversation, and even **to renew their friendship. The code** here is to **show interest in the other person. The way** to do so is as follows: An open smile, a curious look, eye contact, speaking the friend's name and asking after his welfare. A pair chosen by the facilitator performs this meeting as the other group members observe and write down their comments. The pair is followed by the next couple, and the group again writes down its notes in the journals. A discussion is then held in the group forum as the observers share with the pairs that performed what they understood and the facilitator then summarizes the exercise.

EXPERIENCE C – GETTING ACQUAINTED, CREATING RECIPROCITY AND COOPERATION

Two students who have never met before get together to see if they can study with each other for exams. **The task** - creating a positive connection. **The codes – respect for others**, openness, flexibility, compromise. **The way** – presenting yourself without being over-modest or arrogant, using suitable language, maintaining a conversation that is positive in nature. In the group forum: Feedback to those performing the exercise from all the group members and a discussion to increase awareness of what took place at this event: Was a positive connection made? Will they be able to cooperate in learning together for exams? The exercise is then repeated with a second pair from the group.

CONCLUSION

A concluding symposium, open discussion, will be held between the group members. The facilitator will lead the discussion toward having the members describe their experiences, conclusions, lessons learned, etc.

THIRD WORKSHOP –
DEVELOPING SOCIAL LIFE SKILLS

Session 1 – Awareness of Social Codes in Everyday Life
(For distribution to the group members)

A. Social Codes (A Sample)

- Initial words of greeting
- How are you? **Listen to the answer.**
- **Do not interrupt** the speaker (even when it is hard not to do so).
- **Show interest** ("It's nice to meet you" or "It's great seeing you after such a long time").
- **Show appreciation** and respect for the other person, and for whoever is different from you ("It's great how you..."; "I really appreciate your coming here").
- **Say 'Thank you'** and indicate **the reason**: For your help, your advice, etc.
- **Be open** to the customs of other cultures (showing interest and acceptance).
- **Put out your hand for a handshake** – when first meeting and when parting.
- **Show support for someone in distress** (a warm hug, encouragement, giving help).
- Admit to having made a mistake.
- **Ask for forgiveness**, if someone felt insulted or misled.
- **Turn to people by their name** if you know it.

- **Respond to a request** whenever possible.
- **Turn down** a request honestly and tactfully, if you cannot meet it.
- **Direct a social conversation** to a positive pattern and check if **those present** feel comfortable ("I'd like to talk about… Is that okay with you?").
- **Present yourself** to a stranger of your own initiative in a social milieu.
- **Self-humor** - in order to create an open and tension-free atmosphere.
- **Smile** as a sign of personal acquaintance.
- **Check when phoning** if it is a convenient time to talk.
- **Part** with proper words of leave-taking, and not abruptly.
- **When greeting or parting,** do so with a smile and a positive, optimistic tone.
- **The important things** are said at the beginning or at the end of a conversation, or both.
- **Use language that is** appropriate to the situation at hand (a child, a supervisor, etc.)

B. Rules for Engaging in a Flowing Conversation

- **Humor** – general and self-humor and entertaining stories.
- **Active listening** to what is said, to body language, to others' feelings.
- **Obstructive listening** – is pretending, being distracted, seeming bored.
- **Attention to words, gestures** and thinking patterns.
- **Demonstrating self-awareness** – transmits self-confidence, flexibility and openness.
- **Reading body language** to help understand the other per-

son's feelings.

- **Beware of invading** the other person's personal space and privacy, preserve his comfort zone.
- **Eye contact** along with the first handshake of greeting confirms for your dialogue partner your interest in him.
- **Be dressed** appropriately to fit the occasion and increase your confidence and calmness.
- **A hug** demonstrates positive energies. Use this gesture of affection.
- **Social skills can be nurtured** – go for it!!!
- **Avoid being argumentative**, as **winning** an argument is often a social **loss**.
- **Small gestures of friendship** demonstrate caring and develop contact.

THE TASK – PARTICIPATION IS MANDATORY.

a. Contact someone you know, a friend or neighbor, and try to renew your past relationship with him, or try initiating a new relationship with someone you would like to be in contact with. At the group session, the members relate their experiences and the outcome. The group will provide feedback and discuss the dilemmas encountered. (For example: A desire for contact and then withdrawing out of apprehension or concern. What were those concerns? How can they be overcome?). It is important to discuss both the successes and the failures and the members' restraints and examine in depth the less successful events.

b. A joint reading of the list of social codes, with the group discussing each code and together trying to determine its **practical** significance, by raising memories of situations in which they succeeded, failed or were unsure how to conduct themselves in an acceptable manner vis-à-vis their dialogue partner.

The session ends with light conversation over a cup of coffee.

THIRD WORKSHOP – DEVELOPING SOCIAL LIFE SKILLS
Session 2 – Social Codes in Special Situations

INTRODUCTION

All of us at some time have encountered situations in which we are called upon to demonstrate a high sophistication and understanding of social codes. In such cases, both parties are required to proceed with caution, discretion and with the proper application of **intuition**. The major elements of a meeting of this nature are usually empathy and tact. Tactful behavior is based on social understanding and sensitivity. These are sensitive situations in which one of the parties may feel hurt, rejected and frustrated. Therefore, **understanding the context** of the conversation is necessary, as is understanding to what degree a positive connection between the parties is important to each of them. Beyond that, **self-awareness** and understanding social rules and norms are of help in finding the right path. The following three examples, chosen for the experiential exercises, are but samples out of a wide and varied choice of possibilities.

EXPERIENCE A – DEMONSTRATING SUPPORT

The facilitator: 'Bob meets his neighbor, who seems a bit down, and asks how he is. The neighbor replies that he's lost his job, he was fired, and he has four kids and his wife just underwent complex surgery and her recovery is slow, and as a result he's deeply in debt.'

The group members are asked to write in their journals how they would react. Then the facilitator asks for two volunteers to role-play the two neighbors. The other group members receive written instructions as to what they should observe and expect: Was support expressed verbally or via physical gestures? Are they talking to one another openly? In what ways was help offered? The group members write down additional comments and suggestions, and the facilitator then initiates a short discussion.

EXPERIENCE B – TURNING DOWN A REQUEST

The facilitator: 'Joe is a high school student who lives on Dan's block. He heard that Dan is an outstanding student. One day, Joe knocks at Dan's door and asks to speak with him. Dan invites him in and listens to Joe's request to help him prepare for his matriculation exams. However, Dan is too busy and is unable to do so. How will he go about turning him down?'

The facilitator chooses two group members to present the above situation. They do so twice, switching roles: The one playing "Joe" will then play the "student, Dan" who turns down the request, and vice-versa. However, Dan surprises Joe with a totally unexpected request of his own. Even though Joe is just sixteen-and-a-half years old, Dan offers him payment for his help three hours a day in the afternoons, looking after Dan's bedridden grandmother. (To the facilitator: Joe the high school student doesn't know what kind of request he will need to face, as Dan will be getting it secretly in writing.) This time, the person role-playing Joe will have to cope with the surprise factor. Joe is to be prompted in advance, without knowing the details, that he is to turn down Dan's request.

During this role-playing demonstration, the other group members write down their own versions of how they would refuse, as well as comments for the role players.

CONCLUSION

In the group forum, each of the role-players will describe his experience and especially what and how he felt. Then the facilitator will lead a discussion in which the group members voice their suggestions and comments to the performers, and the facilitator together with the group will summarize what has been learned.

EXPERIENCE C – ADMITTING A MISTAKE, APOLOGIZING AND ASKING FORGIVENESS

Facilitator: 'You work at an office in London and you meet Ed at the cafeteria near your office building. Ed studied with you in Junior High School, you always liked him and wanted to keep in touch with him. However, contact with him was lost long ago and you recall that this happened after you had become angry with him and insulted him in front of your classmates. What will you do to renew the connection?'

Each group member writes in his journal what he would say, what gestures he would employ and so on. Then the members read their responses before the entire group.

The facilitator leads a discussion of the various possibilities raised by the group and adds his own suggestions, **only after** all the members of the group have shared their ideas, such as: Explaining what you've been through, admitting a mistake, expressing regret, apologizing, asking to 'forgive and forget' because we were just kids back then, expressing your wish to renew the friendship... and **just as important – at the beginning of the conversation,** asking Ed if he remembers what happened back then and if he is still angry.

CONCLUSION

The question is: Is it possible to turn a new leaf and renew the connection? The emphasis will be placed on the importance of admitting to one's mistake and apologizing, and the accompanying feelings: Embarrassment, shame, regret, relief, satisfaction, etc. The facilitator guides the discussion.

THIRD WORKSHOP –
DEVELOPING SOCIAL LIFE SKILLS

Session 2 – Social Codes in Special Situations
(For distribution to the group members)

At times we are in need of a higher level of sophistication in understanding social codes. In such situations, we need to act with precaution, discretion and staying attuned to our intuition. The major elements are – tactful behavior based on an understanding and sensitivity of what is taking place within the social context and the interpersonal relationships.

Therefore, it is essential to understand the situation in which the conversation is unfolding, the importance of a positive relationship between the parties and, above all, a personal awareness of the sensitivities involved in this relationship. it is also just as important to be able to apply the accepted codes and norms in similar situations.

THE TASK – PARTICIPATION IS MANDATORY.
At this session's meeting, you are asked to describe an event in which you hurt someone else, and regret it. Consult with the other members as to how the damage can be repaired and implemented without hurting someone or being hurt.

Concur on a proposal for changing or correcting what took place.

Discuss those incidents in which you yourself were hurt – what was the nature of the others' attitude that caused you to feel hurt, and how do you feel about it?

How can you amend the feeling of insult that you experienced? How can you repair your relationship with the person who hurt you? With the injured party?

The session ends with light conversation over a cup of coffee.

THIRD WORKSHOP – DEVELOPING SOCIAL LIFE SKILLS
Session 3 – About Belonging and Friendship

INTRODUCTION

First, hold a short discussion about the previous task.

Belonging and friendship are intertwined: both represent basic needs of every human being. The difficulty in creating social ties usually derives from a lack in social skills, which are needed for coping in such situations. This includes difficulty in reading the social map and navigating one's behavior in social situations. These also impact on the ability to develop reciprocal relationships and mutuality. These factors and others are obstacles along the path of helping an initial acquaintanceship develop naturally. Nonetheless, the situation is not irreversible. Through practice with the help of professionals, one can improve his social skills and accomplishments. Forming relationships and maintaining them are a central focus of our lives and without them, other difficulties may arise in other aspects of our lives: in our couple relationship, in the family, with friends, at work or in a social group.

A relationship between friends is based on mutual understanding, empathy and commitment. These conditions facilitate honesty, frankness, acceptance of the other and open communication. In this session, we will actively exercise the process of establishing and basing friendship, in order to improve our skills in this area.

EXPERIENCE A – A CONVERSATION ABOUT FRIENDSHIP

To the facilitator: Encourage a discussion about friendship and try to have all the group members actively involved. Encourage the members to talk about their own experiences. It is important not to pressure those who are unwilling to talk about this subject, which may be painful.

The facilitator should guide the discussion with sensitivity to facilitate openness, enable feedback and encourage the members to turn to one another and engage in active conversation.

EXPERIENCE B – PERSONALITY TRAITS THAT HELP FOSTER FRIENDSHIP

To the facilitator: This exercise is meant to strengthen awareness of those personality traits that help to create a greater closeness with others. A positive ambiance is mandatory for carrying out the exercises related to closeness, mutuality, friendship and belonging.

Each member reads aloud from his journal at least one trait that can improve a friendship. The facilitator writes on the board each trait read by the group members, without noting their names, under the title "Our Pool of Positive Traits." Every trait that re-appears receives an asterisk. The next stage is to relate to the list on the board and discuss the potential of these traits to reinforce social skills. The facilitator asks of each member to choose those traits he would like to adopt, both from the list on the board and other lists.

The facilitator encourages an active discussion between the members and guides them.

Remain aware of any tendency to deviate from the positive direction of the criticism and help as needed.

EXPERIENCE C – ABOUT BELONGING

A discussion of the group forum on the concept of "belonging": Why is it important to belong? What prevents us from belonging? What is the significance of belonging for each one of the group members? How can we reinforce our ties of belonging in those frameworks we are connected with? The facilitator invites all the members to express themselves.

Following that, each member shares with the group **an experience** he has had, what and how he felt, what he learned about himself and his friends. The facilitator sums up and adds further interpretations and insights about the significance of feeling that you belong, and invites **responses from the group.**

THIRD WORKSHOP – DEVELOPING SOCIAL LIFE SKILLS
Session 3 – About Belonging and Friendship
(For distribution to the group members)

Belonging and friendship represent **basic** needs of every human being.

- Creating and maintaining contacts plays an important part in our lives, and without them, we will find it hard to maintain other relationships, such as: couples, friends, work and family.
- A friendship relationship is based on mutual understanding, empathy and commitment – which in turn allow for honesty, open communication, frankness and acceptance of the other.
- Difficulty in forming friendships derives usually from a lack of social skills.
- For example, difficulties in reading the social map and navigating one's behavior in social situations will stand in the way of developing reciprocal relationships and mutuality.
- These skills are important to help us open ourselves up naturally and spontaneously to initiating, building and deepening relationships.

THE TASK – PARTICIPATION IS MANDATORY.
Examine yourselves with the help of your parents, siblings and others, and create a list of social relationships which you feel you are part of. After that, score each relationship with your degree of

belonging, from 1 to 5 on the attached diagram (5 is the highest level of belonging, 1 is the lowest).

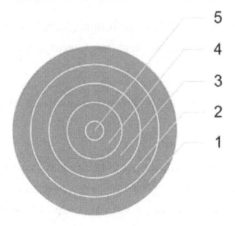

5
4
3
2
1

In the group discussion review the options for reinforcing the contact or the belonging to those frameworks you noted, such as: parents, family, class, social group, neighborhood, country, etc.

Plan in advance to go together to the movies. The organizer will coordinate the time and place that is suitable to everyone in the group and inform the members. Try to choose a film that deals with **the relationships between couples - a pair of friends or a married couple.** How do they maintain the connection between them? What happens when they face a crisis? How do they resolve the crisis positively/negatively? The group can choose to watch a video at one of the members' homes, followed by a discussion over a cup of coffee.

THIRD WORKSHOP –
DEVELOPING SOCIAL LIFE SKILLS

Session 4 – Reciprocity and Personal Space in Friendships

INTRODUCTION

Friendship is based on reciprocity: "I am your friend and you are my friend." We all want to have a friend, but at times we carry unpleasant memories that impact on our desire to maintain social contacts. Many of us yearn for friendships, while others prefer their own company in order to avoid the mental efforts involved in these relationships.

Nonetheless, friends are a source of support and entertainment, they accept you as you are and there is a shared trust, common interests and a desire to share experiences both in good times and bad. Good relationships among friends are not expressed by full agreement between them at all times or on all things. The key to their ongoing relationship is found in the agreement that friends need not think or feel the same way about every topic or in every situation. It is okay not to agree. Good friendship also involves the ability **to understand** the other person's feelings, even without fully identifying with or feeling the way he does. This is the basis for the continuity and deepening of the relationship. Within this "togetherness," it is essential that each one maintains his own personal space that will allow him to be himself. Being friends does not mean being "identical twins," but rather developing a mutual acceptance of one for the other. With time, it is recommended to reach a mutual agreement as to how often you meet, so that each one has his own span of time that he needs to be with himself and his concerns. All of the above-mentioned aspects come under the heading: Personal space in friendship or couple relationships. A friendship does not form of itself. Someone has to initiate it. Such initiative arouses concerns: We are afraid of being rejected and tend to avoid the pain involved in rejection. However, every type of initiative contains the possibility for disappointment. Yet it also contains the potential of hope and a chance. Gaining experience in forming social contacts may strengthen our daring and decrease our apprehension, which in turn will allow us **to take action** instead of **abstention** (progressing instead of regressing). This process begins from the very first encounter. **A well-groomed appearance** and an open smile broadcast a positive attitude. If we smile at people from the beginning, we will create a comfortable ambiance. Active listening and a show of interest in our dialogue partner will increase our chances to succeed. All of these factors will impact on the first impression and most likely on continued contact. When parting with pleasant smiles, light humor and sincere thanks, wishing a good day, success, etc., a positive memory remains and usually leads to a request for continued contact.

EXPERIENCE A – CREATING A FRIENDLY CONTACT

The facilitator asks for a volunteer to the center of the circle. The volunteer spins a bottle, as in the popular childhood game "Spin the Bottle," and approaches the person the bottle pointed at, to invite him to engage in a friendly conversation with him. During this conversation, each one relates about himself whatever he thinks will strengthen the ties of friendship between them. It is important to prepare oneself for active listening and a sincere show of interest of one in the other, and keep in mind that friendship develops on the basis of **honesty and openness.**

The observers sitting in a circle write down their comments. Another group member spins the bottle and initiates a friendly conversation with another partner. This chain of experimentation continues until all members of the group have participated in the exercise. In the meantime, the observers continue writing down comments in their journal. When everyone has had his turn, the facilitator encourages a discussion based on the members' comments regarding the conversations held between the pairs. He then adds his own insights and some tips for leave-taking, such as: "Would you like us to meet again?" "If so, why don't you suggest what's good for you? When? Where? What would you like us to do together?" etc. (The facilitator emphasizes that **it is of utmost importance** to verify what it is the partner wants, and **not to dictate** what you want.)\

EXPERIENCE B – DOING THINGS TOGETHER

The group is divided into threes. One of the three has the role of observer, and the other two have to plan spending time together, including eating out and going to a movie. While discussing this, it becomes clear that each one likes a different movie genre or different kind of restaurant (war films or historic films, a dairy restaurant or fish restaurant, etc.). Nonetheless, they must find a way to spend time together by negotiating, until a solution acceptable to both is reached. Each time they are "stuck," the 'observer' tries to help them or enlists the facilitator.

At the end of the exercise, they are ready with an agreed-upon program, after having checked with the third member (the 'observer') if he too can join them. The group then reports to the group forum how they coped, where they ran into difficulty and how they were helped. The facilitator presents what the typical weak points are, points out the appropriate responses and adds his own insights.

THIRD WORKSHOP – DEVELOPING SOCIAL LIFE SKILLS

Session 4 – Reciprocity and Personal Space in Friendships
(For distribution to the group members)

Friendship is based on reciprocity, but also on **private space** within the friendship.

- A good relationship between friends **is not** always expressed via mutual agreement.
- It is okay not to agree, and good friendship includes the ability to understand the other person's feelings, even if not sharing his feelings.
- Being friends – does not mean being identical twins, but rather to mutually accept one another, with the differences between them.
- With time, it is recommended to reach agreement as to how frequently the friends meet.

A relationship between friends does not form of itself – one of the parties must initiate it.

- The initiative to form contact raises anxiety of possible rejection, and can therefore lead to abstention.
- Gaining experience in forming social ties will strengthen one's boldness and decrease anxiety.
- A certain physical distance creates a comfortable ambiance. A probing manner and intrusive questions create antagonism.

Factors that increase the chances for establishing friendships

The first impression:

- A well-groomed appearance and an open smile broadcast a positive attitude.
- Shaking hands and eye contact.
- Polite remarks, such as "It's nice to meet you," that confirm interest and caring.
- Active listening and demonstrating sincere interest in the other person.

When parting:

Pleasant smiles, light humor and good wishes leave a positive memory in the long run.

THE TASK – PARTICIPATION IS MANDATORY.

The entire group goes to see a movie together, preferably a day show or early evening. The organizer chosen for this task consults with the facilitator to choose a movie that deals with interpersonal relationships, such as: In a class, a group, the family, friends, soldiers in service, a neighborhood gang, etc. Going to a nearby café after the movie for discussion should be planned. The discussion will address: What have we learned from the movie and what can we take from it into our own everyday lives? Did the movie remind us of experiences of ours in the past?

The time planned for this task should be double the usual, to allow for both the film and the ensuing discussion. End with light talk and a cup of coffee, as usual.

THIRD WORKSHOP – DEVELOPING SOCIAL LIFE SKILLS
Session 5 – Preserving and Maintaining a Friendship

INTRODUCTION
Preserving and maintaining a friendship is an ongoing process that consists of a gradual buildup, getting acquainted, deepening the familiarity, connecting, consistent contact, reinforcing the ties, growing closer and preserving stability. No less important is the necessity, when building a friendship, to clarify the differences in personality traits, perspectives, values and customs. Identifying the differences serves to reinforce mutual understanding between the parties and furthers their ability to accept one another.

In this session we will examine the principles and paths of action for preserving and reinforcing friendships.

EXPERIENCE A – FRIENDSHIP AS A PERSONAL NEED
The facilitator encourages the group members to participate in an open discussion about their need for a stable and ongoing friendship. To ascertain that all the members express themselves on this topic, the exercise should be carried out with the group seated in a circle.

Applicable aspirations that will probably be expressed are: Belonging, being understood, cooperation, appreciation, confidence, reinforcing one's self-image, sharing with someone close, meaningfulness, ending a sense of loneliness, etc.

The facilitator will lead a concluding discussion in which the group members are encouraged to share their experiences and hold a meaningful dialogue with the others.

EXPERIENCE B – HELPFUL PERSONALITY TRAITS

Each participant is asked to write down in his journal his own traits and behaviorisms that can be of aid in **connecting** him with others. The objective is to strengthen one's self-awareness in this regard. Each participant reads aloud before the group forum what he has written. These are written on the board and the facilitator asks of the members to share their perceptions as to which traits are helpful and which are hindering. The facilitator encourages everyone to express himself.

The facilitator will organize a **summarizing discussion**, posing the following question: What have I learned about myself and my friends today? How can I utilize what I've learned in my efforts to form friendships or make new friends? Am I capable of correcting or changing my past mistakes?

THIRD WORKSHOP –
DEVELOPING SOCIAL LIFE SKILLS

Session 5 – Preserving and Maintaining a Friendship
(For distribution to the group members)

THE CHARACTERISTICS OF A STABLE FRIENDSHIP

a. Transparency, honesty and reciprocity facilitate behaving naturally, relying on one another, enjoying each other's company and increasing closeness. **Trust is the supporting pillar of a stable friendship.**

b. A relationship that is supportive and accepting nurtures a **desire to continue meeting one another.**

c. Friendship is a relationship that develops over time, from a superficial acquaintance to a deep, extended connection. **Relationships are built and developed.**

d. Superficial relationships are mostly temporary and are maintained on the basis of serving one's interest. **Such relationships do not usually continue to be established or developed.**

e. Long-term friendships are characterized by stability, integrity, commitment, responsibility, openness, trust, acceptance and fondness. In a couple relationship, there are the added facets of **love and intimacy**.

f. A long-term friendship will not fulfill **all the needs** of the individual, but rather will be based on the mutual acceptance that will contribute to understanding and emotional reciprocity.

g. Shared social activities nourish the friendship/couple relationships.

STRATEGIES FOR MAINTAINING FRIENDSHIPS

a. Social abilities and skills are the basis for success. There are several basic social **rules,** such as politeness (expressing thanks, appreciation and respect of others), that are applicable to every situation. There are various behavioral **norms** that one must be familiar with, understand and apply. Both the rules and the norms are usually learned throughout life from interpersonal experiences, or at workshops that develop social life skills.

b. In order to contribute to a primary or ongoing connection, it is important to **employ active listening**. This includes showing interest in the other person, paying sincere attention to him and emphasizing what both parties share in common (such as in the field of studies, a field of special interest, similar experiences, etc.).

c. Confirmation and reinforcement of expressed feelings and emotions (expressing understanding, support and a desire to help, sharing inferences from similar personal experiences).

d. Suggestions for possible solutions out of empathy, while providing details and explanations (and ascertaining that the proposed solution suits the other party).

e. The implementation suggested here is based on the principle of **reciprocity** and will foster the ability to apply and improve the partners' **assertiveness** and their capability to initiate, and even lead, fruitful interpersonal relationships, thus strengthening and maintaining their friendship.

TASK – PARTICIPATION IS MANDATORY

The group meets and reads the above printouts together, pausing on each item for a short discussion. The members are asked to relate their own personal experiences of **success or mishaps**, and engage in a discussion about it with their fellow members.

The session ends with light conversation over a cup of coffee.

THIRD WORKSHOP –
DEVELOPING SOCIAL LIFE SKILLS

Session 6 – Transitions, Changes and Beginnings as Weak Spots

INTRODUCTION

The facilitator opens the session by clarifying the meaning of **transitions, changes and new beginnings**. He describes one or two such experiences he himself has had, to illustrate and normalize the emotional stress that accompanies these situations. Indeed, situations such as these are accompanied by uncertainty, embarrassment, tension and anxiety, as they demand rather complex coping – what was known and familiar is now removed, and what is about to happen remains unclear. Will it be suitable? Will it be disappointing? Etc.

The facilitator asks of the group to give examples of transitional situations, such as: Moving to a new apartment, immigrating to a different culture, beginning a new educational framework, moving from one class to another or from one school to another. All of these, and other situations as well - such as parents' divorce, a death in the family, departing from a close friend – call upon a reorganization of one's abilities to cope.

Emphasis should be placed on the anxieties and doubts that arise during the process of social integration. We ask ourselves: Who are the people that I will meet? Will I find a common language with them? How will I do that? Will they understand me? How will I be received? Who will connect with me and who will reject me? And how will I fit in with the group?

EXPERIENCE A – DISCUSSION AND MUTUAL SHARING

The facilitator asks the group members to recall transitional events from the past and point out the misgivings and difficulties they experienced. He encourages a group discussion, leads the discussion and contributes his own perceptions. He concludes with mentioning different ways of dealing with and alleviating one's distress. When the discussion ends, the facilitator briefly summarizes what has been said.

EXPERIENCE B – LOCATING WEAK SPOTS

The group is divided into threes, each group discusses a problem that comprises two questions, as follows:

Group A:
1. A change in life – How does it demand of me a special coping?
2. What skills/strengths do I possess that I can enlist during the transition period?

Group B:
1. What did I experience during the process of adaptation to our group?
2. What can help me overcome difficulties in social adaptation?

Group C:
1. Which hardship or problem repeatedly arises during beginnings or transitions?
2. How did I manage to overcome a crisis of change in the past?

All three groups choose one member who will write briefly what is said (only the major points). This member is also responsible for keeping the discussion focused and not letting it divert to other topics. The key statement is: "Not for that purpose are we gathered here."

At the next stage a representative of each group will report to the group forum the results of his group's deliberations. The facilitator will gather and summarize the information and give each group feedback on its presentation to the forum.

THIRD WORKSHOP – DEVELOPING SOCIAL LIFE SKILLS

Session 6 – Transitions, Changes and Beginnings as Weak Spots
(For distribution to the group members)

A QUESTIONNAIRE FOR LOCATING WEAK SPOTS (ANSWER IN DETAIL IN YOUR JOURNAL):

1. A change in life – how does it demand of me special coping?
2. What are my strengths which I can enlist during a period of transition?
3. How did I succeed in overcoming a crisis of change in the past? Detail and illustrate.
4. Which difficulties or problems repeatedly arise in situations of beginnings or transition? Detail and illustrate.
5. What did I experience during the period of adaptation to our group?
6. Which new social situations are especially hard for me? Detail and explain.
7. What do I feel can help me overcome difficulties in social adaptation? Detail and illustrate.

TASK – PARTICIPATION IS MANDATORY

The group plans a picnic. Two of the group members take responsibility: one to locate a suitable venue, the second to organize the food. Each group member brings a dish from home and the organizer is responsible to see that the menu is varied, but without exaggeration. Another group member is responsible for the entertainment, bringing something interesting or exciting to read or a subject to discuss.

Good luck!!

THIRD WORKSHOP – DEVELOPING SOCIAL LIFE SKILLS
Session 7 – Fellowship and Friendship

All beginings are hard... do not fear! Cope and be encouraged.

INTRODUCTION

This session focuses on increasing one's awareness and deepening an understanding of the variety of possibilities in social contacts.

The facilitator's opening remarks: An ongoing fellowship that is desirable to both partners may remain as such, but may also flower into friendship and perhaps even to a close relationship. Some of the preconditions for forming a friendly contact include: A pleasant appearance, presenting a good mood and applying the rules for connecting. Self presentation is of special importance and constitutes our "calling card." All these factors together have a decisive impact on the other party in our encounter, as well as on the quality of the ensuing conversation. Ties of friendship call for greater commitment than do the ties of fellowship. The saying, "All beginnings are hard" expresses what all of us experience when we are about to meet someone new. One of the greatest apprehensions that people have in these situations is the concern that they may say, suggest or do **the wrong thing** and subsequently be rejected. Those who have experienced exclusion or social rejection will have greater concerns that may at times be accompanied by anxieties.

EXPERIENCE A – PRACTICAL TOOLS TO DEAL WITH THE PROCESS OF BUILDING FRIENDSHIPS

Following are a number of tips that will help overcome the fear of social failure:

To the facilitator: The list is to be read aloud, pausing on each item for a short discussion to clarify and illustrate it, and encourage the group members to relate their own experiences, both successful and disappointing. It is important that every member express himself.

a. **Paying attention to first impressions**, such as: one's appearance, eye contact, a sturdy, comfortable handshake, a smile and a good mood.

b. **Self presentation** – This calls for preparation in advance, with the general idea and character of your "calling card" to be well planned.

c. **Awareness of body language** –imparting erect posture, confidence **and interest in the other person.**

d. **Demonstrating sincere interest** in the personal history and life of the person we meet, in a relaxed and stress-free manner.

e. **Sense of humor** and the ability to laugh and smile easily, and to relate to yourselves from different angles.

f. **Raising memories** of unique and exciting episodes from your own past or that you witnessed. These will arouse the listener's curiosity and perhaps remind him of similar events. This helps develop a friendly conversation.

g. Use your **active listening skills** and reading body language. Try to remember to mention the names of people who are familiar to you both, if possible.

h.   Try to introduce into the conversation **special contents** that are unique and relate to positive experiences, such as: a great vacation, an excellent film, a sports event, etc. It presents an opportunity for you to reveal excitement.

i.   **Parting with a smile**, a handshake and a good mood. Additionally, a reminder of further contact in the future: Would you like to meet again? Where can we meet? What would you like to do together? Ask your partner what suits him best, **before** stating what you would prefer.

EXPERIENCE B – PLANNING A SOCIAL ENCOUNTER

The facilitator distributes to the group members a printout of the above list of practical tools. He then asks that each participant prepare an outline of what he plans to do when he meets with a friend, and to memorize in detail what he has written in his journal. No one reveals his program to the others. At this stage, the group is divided into pairs and each pair decides on the venue of their meeting (of the exercise): a private home, a party, a group gathering, a club, the workplace, etc.). Each pair demonstrates in front of the group forum a befriending conversation and the observers make notes in their journals. The facilitator helps stage the scenes in which these conversations are played out. After all the pairs have completed their presentations the group forum gathers to provide feedback and comments on each of the presentations.

SUMMARY

What have we acquired in our experiential process today that we can carry with us into our daily lives and utilize? What is easier and what is harder or more complicated? How will we cope?

All the group members in turn express their thoughts. The facilitator relates to the group's experiences and to its process of development, and sums up the exercise.

THIRD WORKSHOP –
DEVELOPING SOCIAL LIFE SKILLS
Session 7 – Fellowship and Friendship
(For distribution to the group members)

Many people are anxious that they may say or do the wrong thing during their first encounter with someone else and subsequently be rejected.

The preconditions for forming a friendly contact include:

- A pleasant appearance and presenting a good mood.
- Applying the rules for connecting.
- Self presentation that suits the occasion.

PRACTICAL TOOLS FOR DEALING WITH THE PROCESS OF BUILDING FRIENDSHIPS

a. Paying attention to first impressions: one's appearance, eye contact, etc.

b. Self presentation – after preparation in advance of your "calling card."

c. Awareness of body language – imparting confidence and interest in the other person.

d. Demonstrating sincere interest in the personal history of our dialogue partner.

e. A sense of humor and the ability to laugh at ourselves.

f. Raising memories of unique and exciting episodes from our past.

g. Active listening skills.

h.   Introducing into the conversation special contents.

i.   Parting with a smile, a handshake and a good mood. And also a reminder of further contact in the future.

TASK – PARTICIPATION IS MANDATORY

- Meet with another member of the group to spend fun time together. **Attendance is mandatory.**

- During the first part of the meeting, the two members hold a personal conversation in a quiet venue (at a café, a private home, the park, etc.).

- The objective of the conversation is to discover what both have in common: shared interests (hobbies, music, sports, etc.). Also, finding a common trait they share, be it in their manner of thinking, their opinions on various topics, etc.

- The conversation should last for about an hour, followed by the entertainment part - going to a movie together, to a club, etc.

Enjoy yourselves!

THIRD WORKSHOP –
DEVELOPING SOCIAL LIFE SKILLS
Session 8 – Relationships and Closeness

INTRODUCTION

In any **long-term** relationship there is closeness to some degree or another. This type of relationship is based first and foremost on reciprocity, which is the 'acid test' of an ongoing relationship. **Reciprocity** is the **central** challenge in a partnership or friendship. It maintains the fabric of friendship and closeness. Deepening the relationship will develop **emotional** reciprocity, which is the giving and receiving of support, encouragement, fondness and acceptance. All this is based, first and foremost, on the **trust** between the parties. Against this background, cooperation and reciprocity can blossom. The qualities of ongoing friendships depend on the above factors in their entirety, and on the feeling that there is mutual enrichment as well.

Among those factors that may be burdensome to a friendship is **frankness**, which grows out of the innocent intention "to tell the whole truth." This will happen when we find it hard to filter and moderate our words. A friend or partner that is nurturing a relationship seeks what **best serves both parties.** He will focus on his partner's strong points and relay a sense of trust and thus will foster stronger ties. On the other hand, repeated criticism may weaken the trust and closeness.

When the partner in a friends' relationship can contain, understand and be respectful of the other partner's uniqueness, the communication between them will bestow calm and comfort and will contribute to greater closeness.

EXPERIENCE A – HOW FRIENDSHIP AND CLOSENESS CAN BE IMPROVED

The group is divided into threes: Each group does some brainstorming and writes down all their thoughts and ideas as to what can set in motion a **positive and long-lasting** relationship.

Then the group forum meets and discusses the suggestions raised. The facilitator helps by writing on the board a summary of these suggestions and each member copies them into his journal.

EXPERIENCE B – SURVIVAL

The **entire** group "sails" to the Caribbean Islands: During the voyage, the boat begins to sink, and everyone in the group manages to swim safely to a nearby shore of an isolated island. The 'survivors' rest on the beach and dry their clothes, as darkness begins to fall. **The group** spends the evening in an attempt **to plan** how they organize themselves for the next morning, to search for shelter and food that will allow them to survive.

In the concluding discussion, the facilitator describes the processes, interactions and decision-making process he noticed during the discussions. He also suggests further insights. The group members respond and he encourages a live discussion on how relationships develop against a background of distress and survival.

THIRD WORKSHOP –
DEVELOPING SOCIAL LIFE SKILLS

Session 8 – Relationships and Closeness
(For distribution to the group members)

a. A **long-term** relationship is based first and foremost on **reciprocity**. It maintains the fabric of friendship and closeness.

b. **Emotional** reciprocity is expressed through the giving and receiving of support, encouragement, fondness and acceptance.

c. **Mutual trust** is the basis and foundation upon which reciprocal growth, enrichment and stable ties can develop.

d. A friend or partner that is fostering a relationship seeks what **best serves both parties** and demonstrates faith in his partner's strong points, is consistent in keeping in touch and in taking responsibility.

e. A critical friend or naïve partner who tells 'the whole truth' directly to his mate, and finds it hard to filter and moderate his words, may destabilize their relationship, because repeated criticism causes embarrassment and unpleasantness to the other party and distances him.

f. When each partner can contain, or tries to contain, the other person,, their mutual feelings of calm and comfort will increase and strengthen the closeness between them.

g. A reciprocal use of feedback, especially for clarifying misunderstandings, reinforces the relationship for the long-term.

TASK – PARTICIPATION IS MANDATORY.

One of the participants prepares a video film to be screened at his home and invites all the group members. The film should deal with the subject of **friendship!!!** The group holds a discussion about the film when it ends, and while it is being screened.

The host prepares refreshments - coffee and cake.

Enjoy yourselves and connect with one another!

THIRD WORKSHOP –
DEVELOPING SOCIAL LIFE SKILLS
Session 9 – A Joint Group Learning Experience
(This session can be scheduled to suit the date of the show that is chosen)

INTRODUCTION

To the facilitator: The experience that was found to be suitable to the learning process in our workshop was a play chosen to reflect the content of this workshop via a story about friendship.

A meeting for a preliminary discussion before attending the play is set for about an hour before the play begins and is held in a café close to the theater. The assumption is that the facilitator has read the book and seen the play. Another get-together is held after the play and is dedicated to a **concluding discussion**. It is important that the group members express their feelings and impressions of the play. The facilitator enriches the discussion and emphasizes those issues that are related to the workshop. The summarizing report should contain the comments of the group members, and will serve to help draw relevant conclusions.

All the above instructions relate to the specific play. If possible, this should be repeated, or another play should be found that deals with friendships in general and the development of long-term relationships in particular. The reactions of the facilitators and the group members significantly contribute to the exemplification and internalization of the contents of the workshop. A search should be done to find and examine every play that addresses the issues of **friendships or couple relationships**. If no such play is available, the group should attend another play that deals with relationships within the family, at work, etc., **depending on the plays** that are running at the time. The plays chosen in the past were:

TASK – MANDATORY
Each group member writes in his journal what he experienced during the play – feelings, memories and insights that surfaced, etc.

THIRD WORKSHOP –
DEVELOPING SOCIAL LIFE SKILLS

Sessions 10 and 11 – Individual Meetings with the Facilitator

Each of these sessions will be dedicated to individual meetings with every member of the group. In every such meeting, the participant will talk in private with the facilitator. Each meeting will last for thirty minutes, during which time the facilitator will encourage the participant to talk, and will listen to his hidden-most feelings. He will also help each one express what he feels and thinks about what was learned in the workshops. Does he feel that in some areas things have changed for him, etc.

It is recommended to check with each participant that he has no objection to the facilitator writing down notes as he speaks.

 In a meeting of this nature, the group member contributes through his personal summing up what he has gained and what needs improvement, thus helping the facilitator learn from him.

Half of the group members will be scheduled to meet during the tenth session and the second half during the eleventh session.

Good luck!

THIRD WORKSHOP –
DEVELOPING SOCIAL LIFE SKILLS
Session 12 – Summing Up and Leave Taking

INTRODUCTION

Today we have reached the end of our joint journey and this is the time to deal with a summing up of what we have been through together in this workshop, what are the conclusions you've drawn from what was learned and considering together how to continue the contact between you.

A. SUMMING UP

We began by working on the basic social skills. These included defining, perceiving and naming our emotions. These are the primary tools for understanding our emotions, i.e., knowing how to define for myself **what it is that I am feeling**, in order to understand **what the other person is feeling**. Following that, we dealt with reading non-verbal language, that is, acquiring skills, observing and understanding what transpires in the mind of another person, beyond verbal communication. We have learned to look directly at our dialogue partner and create eye contact, read facial expressions and understand the significance of the positions and movements of the body and limbs. We emphasized the importance of paying attention to non-verbal cues, in order to decipher their meaning in regard to emotions, thoughts and intentions.

In the second section of the workshop we dealt with skills in interpersonal communication and examined it in various situations. We began by working on active listening skills and continued with exercises on how to engage in a conversation that promotes effective communication and creates contact. We continued on to the next part that addressed the effective management of anger, confrontations and their resolution. Additionally, we dealt with self-advocacy, which was examined as a tool for coping and which comprises the application of all the skills we had learned previous to it.

The last part, which we are terminating today, dealt with developing relationships of friendship. We learned social codes and delved more deeply into understanding social belonging, reciprocity and the maintenance of friendships. We defined fellowship and friendship, as well as relationships and closeness. Together, we viewed films and shows about these topics, which served as tools to further deepen our learning process.

B. INDIVIDUAL SUMMING UP DISCUSSION

Each member is asked to sum up his personal experience: What has he received, what is he taking with him into his everyday life, what is important for him to receive beyond the things we worked on, what are his ambitions and goals for his future and how can they be fostered.

An opinion about the workshops, including feedback for the facilitators, will be welcomed.

To the facilitator: Undeniably, it is important to give the group feedback and describe the process the participants went through via the group experience, and the trust, consolidation and mutual support that were created.

The facilitator then recommends **meeting once a month** on a set day – for example, the first Sunday of every month, or something similar. Suggest that the group members take upon themselves to remind each other anew each month, with each member in turn being responsible for one meeting.

The session ends with words of parting and best wishes for the future.

The group members will give each other short letters, which contain personal feedback **for each one** of the participants. The letters will focus on the strengths that should be utilized and the weak points that should be improved.

It is recommended to encourage both individual and group get-togethers and, **follow-up meetings** with the facilitator. These are important, interesting and educational, and are definitely worth maintaining.

PART IV

INTEGRATING INTO THE COMMUNITY
AND SELF-FULFILLMENT

I – SUITABLE EMPLOYMENT

CHAPTER 1: ASPERGER'S (ASD) AND THE CHALLENGE OF EMPLOYMENT

Venturing and doing are the doors to the hall of success.

INTRODUCTION

Adults with Asperger's (ASD) define their abilities in relation to their career or employment as measured against their success or failure in that field. Attwood (2007) comments that the number of those employed for the long-term is relatively small, and that a lack of success in one's career is one of the causes of depression in this population.

Grandin and Duffy (2004) note that without employment, an unhealthy situation arises for both the individual and society, as these individuals consequently live in isolation, with the syndrome navigating their life. Society loses out on the potential contributions of these talented people and they, for their part, lose the opportunity of enjoying social contact with their colleagues, and remain without a framework they can belong to, and without self-fulfillment.

Fast et al. (2004) in their book present a collection of individual stories, as related to them by adults with Asperger's (ASD), who were diagnosed after having searched for their way for many years. The stories reflect their shared difficulties derived from their syndrome and the differences between them, also emphasizing the uniqueness of each one. During their childhood, they were different from their social environment and as adults it was hard for them to find their place in the field of employment. This resulted from their difficulties in adjusting to a framework and their deficiencies in human relations skills, despite their having worked with aptitude and diligence. Most of them have a hard time coping with competition, authority figures and conflicting situations.

Apparently there are two major factors that critically impact on the success in one's career, for the adult with Asperger's (ASD), and the reciprocal relationship between them: **The first factor** is the crucial difference between a benevolent, accepting and supportive work milieu, which promotes growth and prosperity, and a rejecting and hostile milieu. **The second factor** is the ability of adults with Asperger's (ASD) to apply their intelligence in order to identify the field of employment most suitable to them, yet they find it hard to initiate and demonstrate assertiveness, etc.

It seems that most of those employed find themselves in jobs that do not require special skills and they earn very low pay. This is especially surprising, in view of the fact that many of them have no problem learning and have completed a university education. In contrast, studies indicate frequent mood swings commonly found among these adults, and a significant degree of depression. One possible explanation is the lack of suitable employment and a void of fitting social activities. This leads to an impoverished quality of life, deriving from a constant existential sense of social exclusion and a life of loneliness.

The required social-communal support is:

a. Expanding the awareness and understanding of the syndrome.

b. Expanding accessibility to diagnosis of the syndrome and

      improving accessibility to services that help prepare for an independent life within the community.

c.   Improving the compatibility of professional training to one's career.

d.   Developing suitable programs of the Employment Bureau.

e.   Implementing placement at workplaces that facilitate the adults' adjustment and perseverance.

f.   Investing in imbuing social confidence and skills for an independent life, and addressing issues such as managing emotions, functional behavior, etc.

g.   Developing social skills.

A PROGRAM FOR SUPPORTIVE EMPLOYMENT

In Great Britain there are a number of programs for supportive employment, planned jointly with the National Autism Organization. This project offers a flexible package of pre-employment training, which includes communication skills at the workplace, searching for employment, writing a curriculum vita, qualifications for succeeding in a job interview, awareness of one's limitations and choosing suitable employment.

As one begins working, he is escorted on a daily basis by a fellow worker who serves as his mentor for a two-to-four-week period, with a steady decrease in escorting over that time period. The mentor sees to it that the new employee learns and understands the social as well as occupational demands of his job. He also advises the employers how to cope with problems that arise. In addition, meetings are held regularly between the mentor and the department head. Studies prove that a person with Asperger's (ASD) is definitely capable of fulfilling his job in a full-time position, with the proper support. Moreover, all existing programs should include pre-employment training and individual support, which contribute toward building self-confidence. It is further recommended that social events be organized, **outside** the employment program, to fortify social skills. It is important to understand that this also contributes to one's performance at work, for if the social skills find a venue of expression, then most likely **the feeling of satisfaction at work will increase.**

Adults with Asperger's (ASD) usually tend to lose their jobs due to problems in the area of interpersonal communication, such as misunderstanding social norms, authoritative relationships, etc.

Three issues have been identified as potential trouble spots in the workplace: Issues related to society and communication, issues regarding planning and flexibility, and sensory issues. Clearly, adults with Asperger's (ASD) need a mentor at their workplace who will help them as needed. Researchers emphasize the importance of **preparing the fellow workers of the employee with the syndrome, by familiarizing them with his difficulties and thus enabling them to help him with his social and communication problems.**

In conclusion: It is noteworthy that a large proportion of adults with Asperger's (ASD) function at a high level and have acquired a university education, yet despite their abilities, the unemployment rate among them is high. This situation has a crucial impact on their quality of life, mental health and independence. Therefore, top priority should be given in making the employment market more accessible to them. In addition, supportive programs should be integrated that include, among other things, groundwork preparation of the employers to ensure that the candidates receive personal adjustments in their workplace, suited to the individual needs.

OCCUPATIONAL REHABILITATION

Young people with Asperger's (ASD) demonstrate an ability for higher learning, but many of them carry a history of failed attempts to adjust to occupational frameworks.

An **engineer** with Asperger's (ASD) was offered a position at a technical plant. To the best of his understanding, he was slated for a position dealing with diagnosing and correcting problems that arose. To his surprise, he found himself placed to work on an assembly line. Even though he had superb technical and implementation skills and a tendency toward precision, he was fired on the contention that he works too slowly, thus harming the assembly line's production.

Today, there is greater awareness taking root of the need to create friendly workplaces in the community, for people who are physically and mentally challenged. Employment advisors are trained in evaluating the professional abilities and adjustment problems for each individual. This orientation requires economic resources and hopefully it will expand and prove its worthiness.

Fast et al. (2004) point out that many of the adults with Asperger's (ASD) report that their counselors tend to think their failures resulted from a negative attitude or personal problems and not from the syndrome. This outlook reflects the gap between the need for employment coaches especially trained to escort the rehabilitation process, and their availability.

The perception that occupational rehabilitation should focus on the individual and on placement in a friendly workplace raises the need for training consultants and various support and escorting personnel who are willing to study in depth about Asperger's (ASD) and its consequences. In addition, there is need for a unique rehabilitation framework for adults, which will gather the accumulative knowledge and experience in regard to developing social life skills and providing tools for coping with the challenge of employment at all stages.

Fast concludes that all occupational rehabilitation personnel and employment advisors must understand the unique limitations of adults with Asperger's (ASD) and how these impact on the potentially rehabilitated adults. Meyer (2001) warns that those involved will not be able to help them without understanding the limitations and skills of each one of them.

I – SUITABLE EMPLOYMENT
CHAPTER 2: THE OCCUPATIONAL ROUTE

Only a relatively small number of adults with Asperger's (ASD) are employed in long-term positions suitable to their intellectual abilities and professional skills. The situation is created in which their potential talents are not realized, even though our society needs the advantages and qualities that people with the syndrome have to offer. Conversely, for those diagnosed with Asperger's (ASD), their career is a central, crucial factor in forming their self-identity. The conditions of their work environment and human relations constitute a significant contribution to this process. Adults with Asperger's (ASD) need special preparation toward their occupational life and it should begin as early as possible. Diagnosis and occupational training are an important basis in the preparation process, even before these adults have been trained in a specific field.

However, the unique and focal issue of training for the work-force, shared in common by those adults who have had past training and experience, is the social and interpersonal factor. Accumulative clinical experience indicates that this is their Achilles' heel in adjusting to their place of work. Based on this assumption, a preparatory program should be designed that accompanies the occupational channel, to be implemented regularly in a progressive sequence, for the duration of the rehabilitation program.

THE SOCIAL CHANNEL – THE OPENING WORKSHOP

This channel, as its name implies, is about the relationships between people from different perspectives, which employs a variety of methods (see the section on Workshops for Developing Social Life Skills). This framework enables the participants, youth and adults with Asperger's (ASD), to share a social experience in a controlled environment. For a person with the syndrome a social experience is a special event, therefore it is fitting to say that for him, "One experience is worth a thousand pictures." The group process is led by a skilled facilitator, with expertise in working with special populations. It is important that the facilitator understand the unique difficulties of adults with Asperger's (ASD) and its complexities. This is a group experience under controlled conditions, in which the participants learn how to improve their human relations skills. It is carried out under protected conditions that facilitate effective learning, led by an expert facilitator.

What has been learned is then implemented in the everyday life of each participant in his natural surroundings. In this way, new opportunities are open to him to connect, to feel that he belongs, to build friendships and improve his human relations skills.

FIRST STAGE – CONSOLIDATING FIELDS OF OCCUPATION

In this stage, each of the participants will personally deal with consolidating his needs and skills, and may include occupational diagnosis for whoever needs it. This stage will be relevant especially for the young adults with Asperger's (ASD) who are in the program.

At the same time, the group of adults and those with past employment experience will participate in a workshop for occupational self-awareness, which will contend with identifying, defining and internalizing the various causes of the hardships and failures in their past employment venues, and will reinforce their awareness of their talents and skills.

SECOND STAGE – BECOMING FAMILIAR WITH THE AREA, OR A REALITY CHECK

During the sessions devoted to this topic, tours will be conducted of the workplaces relevant to the desired employment for the group members.

The tours will be conducted for the entire group, sub-groups or individuals. They will enable the adults with the syndrome to test their suitability to the work environment - from its physical aspects (noise, crowdedness, etc.), its human environment and from the perspective of a large, divergent organization compared to a small firm. All this will later be processed via group discussions with the facilitator. At the end of this stage, it is expected that the participants in the rehabilitation program will be integrated into practical employment in these workplaces, or in others that are suited to them.

THIRD STAGE – PRACTICAL WORK

In this stage, the participants will be placed in part-time or temporary employment, and an escorting mentor will prepare the employers and colleagues, as well as guide and mediate between the parties.

The group will meet once a week for a discussion to process experiences and difficulties at work, with the help of the mentor. At the end of this stage, conclusions will be drawn with the group members and practical plans will be formed for implementation at work.

FOURTH STAGE – PREPARATION FOR OCCUPATIONAL PLACEMENT

At this stage, a workshop will be held that deals with life skills, focusing on preparations toward the process of looking for employment and successful integration at the workplace. The workshop will address issues of personal grooming, organizing time, understanding organizational structure, team relationships, authoritarian relationships, thinking along lines of planning and implementation, organizing information and preparing for a job interview.

FIFTH STAGE – LOOKING FOR EMPLOYMENT AND ACTUAL PLACEMENT

This stage will focus individually on each group member in the rehabilitation process. The placement personnel, who have specialized in the rehabilitation of adults with Asperger's (ASD), will track down potential workplaces. They will work intensively to prepare these frameworks and encourage a benevolent, supportive and accepting environment.

At the same time, each of the rehabilitants will be asked to research the workforce in his own field or profession and in his geographical area. The results will be submitted in writing and a discussion of all the steps to be taken will be held before beginning work, and how to apply the skills in organizational management, based on the principles learned in the rehabilitation program.

PROGRAMS FOR OCCUPATIONAL SUPPORT

There are two categories of occupational support: One employs the view of pre-occupational training, whereas the other proposes support within the employment framework from the moment the new employee begins his job.

The first method employs a holistic approach, thus the focus on preparation for employment is not solely on occupational skills. It includes help in developing social confidence and skills for independent living, to promote knowledge and independence that will enable success.

Additionally, training is invested in topics such as managing emotions, strategies for planning and coping in everyday life, as well as organizing group outings and entertainment to encourage social experience.

There are projects that are involved in volunteer occupational placement, in order to develop skills related to success at work, in preparation for future employment.

Pre-occupational training includes: Communication skills at the workplace, seeking a position and consultation in choosing a suitable occupation. As soon as employment begins, the new employee is accompanied by a full-time mentor, for the first four weeks of employment. It is his responsibility to assure that the new employee understand the social and professional requirements related to his job. He advises him how to deal with problems that arise and how to avoid their occurrence. The mentor holds regular meetings with the employee's supervisor. There are programs that provide ongoing support for full-time workers.

In a follow-up study that compared adults who were employed in a sheltered framework to another group employed within the community, no differences were found in the autistic symptoms between the two groups. On the other hand, in a **five-year follow-up, there was a significant improvement in the quality of life of those adults employed within the community, compared to those employed in sheltered frameworks. Additionally, most managers reported that the mentors helped to handle**

problems that arose all along the way. The number of hours of support gradually decreased within a period of four months of employment, and accordingly so did the cost, **which led to the employers' agreement to hire more candidates. Thus the accessibility to jobs increased and the number of those who progressed to independent living also increased relatively.**

I – SUITABLE EMPLOYMENT

CHAPTER 3: ISSUES RELATED TO EMPLOYING ADULTS WITH ASPERGER'S (ASD)

INTRODUCTION

This section is targeted at helping various work organizations in the process of absorbing and employing people with Asperger's (ASD) that possess good learning abilities. Most of them are highly motivated to succeed in the professional field they have chosen and in which they are meant to attain achievements. However, their success is reliant on the readiness of senior staff personnel in the organization to help them understand and adjust to the accepted behavior codes. Adults with Asperger's (ASD) are known to make mistakes in the area of interpersonal relations. With the help of patience and tolerance of those around them, mutual trust will increase along with their sense of being accepted. With this feeling, they will be able to react more openly, to recruit their learning abilities and improve those areas they find difficult. As a result, they will be more open to share their talents and best skills at their workplace and the organizations will enjoy optimal production from dedicated and industrious workers.

GENERAL REMARKS

Adults with Asperger's (ASD) find it hard to build a career suited to their abilities, even though they are **talented** and industrious workers. Their most blatant difficulty is in adjusting to the framework, due to social hardships, which include dealing with competition, authority figures, confrontations, etc.

Professional literature presents testimonials that indicate two major factors which have critical impact on the occupational success of a person with the syndrome: The primary factor is the crucial difference between a benevolent, accepting and supporting environment to an intolerant and even hostile environment. A supporting environment leads to the blossoming and thriving of those lucky enough to have integrated into it.

The second factor is the ability of the adult with Asperger's (ASD) to enlist those around him to help him succeed, by applying his intelligence and awareness as to which occupational field suits him best. He therefore needs professional training and social support in all the preparatory stages prior to his employment.

The following are two conditions that help a person with Asperger's (ASD) integrate into the workforce:

a. The presence of a significant figure who helps identify his potential skills.
b. A trainer who helps develop his talents and social (and professional) skills related to his sought-after career.

Thus, emphasis must be placed on the crucial role of close training and escorting suited to the individual needs of each person, during the process of his occupational rehabilitation. In Great Britain and the United States, and in Israel, there is a growing awareness of creating "user-friendly" places of employment within the community, for people with special needs. Occupational rehabilitation workers and mentors at workplaces are learning to get to know and understand the unique difficulties of adults with

Asperger's (ASD), along with their unique abilities, in order to help them succeed in their careers.

A successful placement needs to be carried out at three levels correspondingly, and with the cooperation of all parties:

a. Preparing the framework at the potential workplace.
b. Preparing the future employee.
c. Planning a gradual process in which both sides will learn how to interact with one another.

It is recommended to have the candidate meet with those who will be working alongside him, before he begins his employment. This preliminary meeting and the employer's greater familiarity with the syndrome's characteristics will serve as a basis for mutual cooperation during the new worker's absorption process. At the same time, the preliminary acquaintance with the workplace and staff will contribute to the new worker's sense of familiarity upon beginning his new job. A supportive supervisor or an escorting mentor can help the person with the syndrome correct interpersonal mistakes, such as: How to talk with colleagues and customers, how to react in situations of disagreement without expressing crude criticism, and how to apologize and implement a positive rectification diplomatically. Having the new worker with the syndrome begin his employment in a new place in this manner creates a healthy infrastructure for open communication, which in turn reinforces mutual **trust** and cooperation. All this carries an added value that is indeed priceless: The objective here is to lead the people in the surroundings of the adult with the syndrome show understanding of his "strange" behaviorisms and refrain from judgment, thus increasing the staff's readiness to help him. Supportive colleagues and an open dialogue will encourage the new worker to give his very best, a win-win situation which is to everyone's gain.

People with Asperger's (ASD) usually have several characteristic personality traits which, in themselves, can also contribute positively to their workplace - traits such as: directness, loyalty, reliability and a strong ethical code. All these traits indicate someone with integrity who can be relied upon. Add to these: high-level thinking, motivation, industriousness and diligence, which together provide a further advantage in coping with the challenges of a career **in a supporting environment**. For these reasons, they can become attractive candidates for employment.

From the implementation perspective, the above can be summarized as follows:

a. People diagnosed with Asperger's (ASD) need the clarity and transparency of rules, norms, regulations and definitions. This includes the basic rules of everyday life as well, which should also be clearly presented. Take into consideration that even though they find it hard to understand this intuitively, they will definitely respond affirmatively to clear guidelines, especially in the context of an accepting and supporting environment.

b. For similar reasons, it is important to create a work environment that is well planned and **structured**, and to help them learn the hierarchical structure of the organization and the order of the different stages of work.

c. Adults with Asperger's (ASD) cannot always understand what the other person is thinking or feeling, therefore it is recommended that things be expressed verbally: "I think that… if we do it that way… people will be accepting of it… It will encourage cooperation, the results will be… we will achieve our goal"; "I **feel** comfortable working with you, and I hope you feel the same, working with me," etc.

Adults with the syndrome are pleasant and intelligent people. At the same time, they tend, more so than others, to make mistakes regarding other people, unintentionally. That is, their ability to express disagreement or opposition in tactful, sophisticated ways is not sufficiently developed and therefore what they say is not filtered. Being straightforward and honest people, they "say it like it is" and find it hard to understand where they have gone wrong. This is a very important issue at the workplace and the mentor should and can help them figure out what happened and how they can correct this (apologies or discussion, etc.). If we act on the assumption that there is **a relationship of trust between the worker and his mentor**, this can be a very fruitful learning process, which will create a secure place in which one can **develop and seek advice.**

I – SUITABLE EMPLOYMENT

CHAPTER 4: SOCIAL PROBLEMS AND SOCIAL SKILLS AT WORK

Social rules play a central role in interpersonal relations, however internalizing the proper application of these rules is a sophisticated undertaking that continues throughout life, as noted by Meyer (2010). He adds that social rules are not carried out in a vacuum. The interpersonal experience has endless nuances through which the social rules are implemented, and they cannot all be contained in written instructions.

Many of the adults with Asperger's (ASD) find it difficult to decipher the meanings **beyond** the spoken words, but in fact it is the decoding and application of these rules that define the social skills. In addition, people with the syndrome do not tend to spontaneously check with their dialogue partner what exactly did he mean, whereas effective communication develops out of mutual clarification, through which the parties check and recheck with one another if they both understand **the meaning** of the verbal message.

Since most adults with the syndrome have a difficult time deciphering non-verbal cues and sensing intuitively what others think and feel, and making eye contact, it is hard to build trust. Moreover, there is also a malfunction in thinking and communicating in pragmatic language, which makes it hard for them to understand what their supervisors and colleagues expect of them, and they lack the tools to correct their mistakes. With such social deficiency, it is very hard to maintain informal relationships, to operate freely along the social axis and work through cooperation.

Two significant traits that employers look for in their new employees are flexibility with change and the ability to learn. However, adults with Asperger's (ASD) have a difficult time in new situations. According to Meyer (2001), these situations are too complicated for them, as the work culture of today is, by its very nature, a culture of quick changes. The traits that characterize them, such as reliability, devotion and industriousness, may reinforce one's belief that they can be relied upon. Yet, their limitations in social skills may impact on the considerations of the decision-makers as to whom to hire, whether to continue employing the person or to have him promoted. At times, outstanding workers with the syndrome are fired, as perhaps they were called upon to deal with internal organizational politics and failed. This is a complex social situation for which they lack the proper tools for coping.

The important social skill that must be acquired is understanding the feelings and cues from one's fellow workers. Mood changes must be picked up on, attention given to body language, to passive-aggressive behavior and to finding ways to neutralize anger and concern. It is essential to know how to talk with colleagues and customers, how to react in situations of disagreement without expressing criticism crudely, and to know how to apologize if it happens. The escorting mentor at the workplace can help correct mistakes in the interpersonal field and teach the rules. This is effective mainly when the worker with the syndrome possesses professional talents that are appreciated and contribute to the organization.

Adults with the syndrome tend to point out mistakes and express criticism of their colleagues when such mistakes upset the inherent order of things. In such cases, the mentor can help them and teach them diplomatic behavior. For example, he can teach, demonstrate and practice with them how to give feedback in order to open a channel of communication with positive ambiance. He can point out the mistake made and suggest ways of correcting it.

It is important that adults with the syndrome who are employed realize that the workplace may have directors or managers that are supportive, but there are also those who are authoritative, and the employee must learn how to get along with the latter as well. It is suggested that the employee with the syndrome enlist help from a mentor or fellow workers who know how to support and guide him.

The difference in the manner of thinking is an additional problem, as pointed out by Fast (2004): People with the syndrome perceive the neurotypical person as someone who behaves irrationally, as he does not say exactly what he means and does not pay attention to details. On the other hand, their neurotypical colleagues at work show a lack of understanding of their behavior, which may include isolating themselves during breaks, waving their arms about and rocking their body, etc.

In this regard, the obvious question is whether or not it is possible to train the mind of an adult with the syndrome, in order to change his perception, manner of thinking and behavior vis-à-vis the social world.

Meyer (2001) reports that today it is accepted practice to use methods borrowed from the field of the cognitive rehabilitation of adults. He claims that adults with Asperger's (ASD) report that cognitive behavioral therapy (CBT) has a beneficial influence on them and helps them progress.

From experience with brain-damaged individuals, it is now known that it is possible to rehabilitate a **function** that has been damaged. There are hypotheses regarding everyday language and effective functioning, that claim it is possible to also rehabilitate people who never had that ability. The implications of brain research have already been implemented and there is greater acceptance of the approach of long-term teaching of new skills to adults, to upgrade their quality of life. Cognitive rehabilitation is a tool meant to train adults with Asperger's (ASD) in social skills. **There are things they are capable of changing**, each at his own pace. Many of them are aware of the fact that social skills are essential to their success in their adult life, both in their career and their personal life.

I – SUITABLE EMPLOYMENT

CHAPTER 5: ISSUES IN PLANNING A CAREER AND PREPARATION FOR ENTRY INTO THE WORKFORCE

The distance between the freedom to be and the freedom to do is in the aspiration.

Fast (2004) holds that there are three types of people: Those who **cause** things to happen, those who **observe** and those who **are amazed** by what has taken place. People with Asperger's (ASD) usually fall into the third category, and that is why they need professional help and support from their environment at every stage of preparation toward entering the workforce.

Attwood (2007) claims that the professional help must be based upon the understanding that this syndrome is a phenomenon whose source is in neurological variance. This perception enables us to understand the source of the difficulty, and at the same time to nurture and manifest the talents and abilities of those with the syndrome.

Research shows that adults with the syndrome are capable of succeeding in a variety of occupations after having learned to identify their strong qualities and those that should be reinforced. Grandin and Duffy (2004) emphasize the conditions that were common to those adults with Asperger's (ASD) that enabled them to succeed in integrating into the workforce:

a.   They had trainers who helped them develop both social and professional skills related to the career they sought to develop.

b. There was a significant figure who helped them develop their talents and from an early age provided them with feedback regarding their ambitions and plans, **to prepare them for the future.**

c. They took medications and dietary supplements in order to balance their sensory sensitivities, anxieties and depression.

Meyer (2001) holds that it is possible and necessary to divert the energies spent on apprehensions toward planning and active preparation, starting from discovering and nurturing talents and up to adapting them to the workforce. He recommends a rehabilitative strategy called "person-focused planning." This method is suitable for the rehabilitation of adults with Asperger's (ASD) who find it hard to manage themselves functionally and organizationally, and it helps them develop a faith in themselves and trust in others. Thus they learn to differentiate between their own needs and those of others, which serves to alleviate their introversion and focus on their own progress.

This process includes an examination of the ambitions of the person with the syndrome and taking responsibility for his future. Meyer (2001) claims that to do so requires hard, persistent work, along with a repetitive examination of whether the plans for the future stand the test of reality. Skills in planning, management and organization should lead to greater independence, as well as to organizing tasks, thoughts and time. Fast (ibid) suggests using these tools in order to plan, set priorities, set goals and solve problems.

Training and practice should begin with the development of practical daily skills of meeting schedules, organizing current tasks, seeing to the maintenance of the body, the living environment and work environment. This is **the basis** when thinking in terms of planning and implementing as part of the process of preparation for the workforce and fulfilling the awaited job.

In the next stage, guidance and training should focus on helping the adult with the syndrome recognize, understand, define and communicate his abilities and limitations. This can be done via an effective organization of information, in order to disconnect from just one possibility, to open up to additional options and understand the final outcome. It is therefore important to develop a didactic program that will address all these elements, in order to develop skills of self-management, organization and implementation.

These processes will help the adult with the syndrome to better understand his tendencies, ambitions and plans. He will thus learn to calculate alleviating factors against hindrances and reach more correct decisions. Along with that, thought should be given to his fields of interest, his talents, skills, mood, values and personality – what helps him and which activities contribute to him.

This perception is based on the approach, "The person is at the center." imbuing him with the ability for self-definition based on his strengths, which also includes an understanding of the challenging factors. An additional link is intensive work with the counselor on strategies, adjustments, ways of adaptation and tools with which he can change or improve whatever is possible.

An additional advantage is individual development and self-awareness, especially if it is the outcome of a comprehensive training program for employment, targeted at people with Asperger's (ASD), and on condition that it is carried out by professionals specializing in rehabilitating adults with this syndrome.

Fast (2004) suggests a model that compares strengths against weaknesses according to four categories: Cognitive, emotional, social and communicative. With the many social problems that exist in all areas of employment, the candidate's work will lean on **his strengths in a flexible and encouraging work environment**.

It is important that adults with Asperger's (ASD) be familiar with the employment market in their area of education, profession, skills and expertise. Therefore, every person in rehabilitation should be encouraged to search and discover what exists in the work market in his field. The results of his search will be compared to what is desired and what is available.

A written summary of these processes is of the greatest importance, from which several conclusions can be drawn:

a. The effectiveness of the method for preparing the candidate for job placement.

b. Did the approach of "The person is in the center" contribute to the cooperative teamwork of the caregivers and escorts?

c. Did this approach empower the candidate and enable his preparation for placement to his satisfaction?

d. Was what he had experienced and learned reflected in his optimal placement and in a manner of functioning suited to him during his employment?

I – SUITABLE EMPLOYMENT
CHAPTER 6: THE PROCESS OF PREPARING A FACILITATING, SUPPORTIVE WORKPLACE

The strategy that is at the heart of the rehabilitative approach for adults with Asperger's (ASD) is based on professional and functional training toward the transition into a life of regular employment. This is a long process. Additionally, locating the proper placement that suits the skills and education of the adult with Asperger's (ASD), as well as finding a workplace that will be open to accept and absorb him, is also a long and complex process. Therefore, it is preferable to carry out both processes simultaneously.

The first objective is **identifying places** that are reasonably suited to the needs and abilities of the person in rehabilitation – this includes locating employers in the matching fields, and having the placement coordinator visit the organizations and familiarize himself with them.

The second objective is an in-depth examination of the potential workplaces, which includes examining the physical conditions and the readiness of the executive personnel and the staff to be accommodating, accepting and receptive of someone different, etc.

The third objective is **preparing the candidate** for the job. This preparation includes both individual and group work on the accepted rules of human relations at the workplace, becoming familiar with its organizational structure, its authority figures and other relevant characteristics.

The fourth objective is **providing the necessary skills** for the candidate's successful acceptance to the desired position. This includes preparing a curriculum vita and accompanying documents, practice through simulating job interviews, self-advocacy, etc.

As to the matter of the candidate's honest disclosure about his syndrome, when and how it should be done needs to be examined. Usually, the candidate himself should raise this matter during his self-advocacy presentation – which calls for preparing him, as well as the employer, toward this step.

The fifth objective is **an introductory meeting** between the candidate who was hired and his colleagues at work. The importance of this meeting lies in its reducing the candidate's anxiety from the new situation, as already on his first day at work, the adult with Asperger's (ASD) will be encountering people who are familiar to him. In this regard, attention should be given to one's self-advocacy and the counselor should practice with him how to introduce himself and his skills, abilities and talents.

The sixth objective is to **involve the executives** and colleagues of the candidate with Asperger's (ASD) in his social and professional absorption. This includes preparing the staff, through a lecture and discussion with a specialist in occupational rehabilitation of adults with Asperger's (ASD). Such a forum will enable everyone to process the change together, acquire insights and internalize the importance of cooperation in the absorption process of the new employee with special needs.

The seventh objective is **escorting the new employee** for a predetermined time period, with maximum accessibility to the mentor who provides guidance, support and mediation. This accessibility will decrease gradually with time. The mentor's "open door" is of great importance, after the escorting period as well, as it will give the rehabilitated worker someone to turn to in his hour of need.

The eighth objective is **encouraging mutual understanding** and cooperation between the employer and the mentor. This includes executing the organization's modes of action, such as: Encouraging the employee to be responsible and conduct himself according to the policies of the workplace, while demonstrating his willingness to learn its behavioral codes and showing a positive, optimistic attitude. Workers with Asperger's (ASD) need an employer who is open to people with special needs and is ready to hire them, suitable to their professional level, and to nurture a friendly work environment.

When a relationship based on trust exists between the employee and his mentor, a secure place is created for the employee to open up and seek advice, relax and learn how to cope in a better way in the future. When his fellow workers are aware that this employee with the syndrome finds it hard to adjust himself, due to his limitations, they will understand that it is they who should adjust themselves to him. They will try to understand the different ways in which he perceives the situation, and thus will encourage understanding between the parties. It is important to understand that the employee with the syndrome does not always understand what to us seems obvious in human relations.

TIPS FOR EMPLOYERS*
COMMUNICATION AND CONTACT

Listen to him until the end with patience, this will empower the employee with the syndrome. If your time is limited, inform him of this in advance.

Ask for an explanation of things that aren't clear to you, before concluding that he isn't making any sense. Thus you will be expressing your willingness to understand him.

Apply your desire to create understanding. Try to connect to what he is experiencing.

Check to ascertain that he fully understands what was said, thus you will reach mutual understanding. The appropriate technique is that each party repeatedly checks with the other party – "Is this what you meant?"

Respect – Giving full and non-judgmental attention to your employee with Asperger's (ASD) leads to a positive start toward fruitful relationships.

Empathy – Try to step into your employee's shoes, his fears and frustrations, and imagine how you would feel in his place. Support accompanied by **empathy and little advice** is the most effective.

Trust - When trust is achieved, communication flows more easily. The employee with the syndrome is more relaxed, his anxiety level decreases and he is open to learning the skills required of him at his job. It is important that your attitude and interaction with him receive positive resonance throughout the organization.

Acceptance – Every adult with the syndrome is unique, even within the spectrum. Therefore time should be devoted to becoming familiar with his insights, thoughts, beliefs and consciousness, which will help him feel that he is accepted.

Advance to a better place by creating a calm atmosphere. This will encourage communication and a comfortable feeling.

Greater acceptance – People with the syndrome experience being misunderstood and not accepted, therefore it is important that their acceptance be done in a clear, explicit manner ("I understand," "I know," "I'm aware of that," etc.). Phrase your feelings as a question ("Are you angry about that?," etc.).

Connecting – Try to create a sense of connection and contact (a handshake, having coffee together, etc.).

Explain in advance in great detail what is expected of the new employee.

Plan ahead, and share your plans with him, to help him understand what is going to happen. Thus he can start his routine work feeling relaxed. The adult with the syndrome feels **relief when he understands what is about to take place.**

Step in When Something Goes Wrong.

Pay Attention to Any Small Signs of Change.

Place before him all the possible options, in order to discuss them.

Emphasize that you are non-judgmental toward him.

Time framework – Be **clear and understood** as to a time framework, mark the halfway marker of the time period toward achieving the goal and its end marker.

Repeat the important things in different ways.

Failure as feedback – We all make mistakes, and they serve as an excellent opportunity for learning. This must be emphasized over again to people with Asperger's (ASD). ("Was the mishap a result of the program, its implementation or the conditions? What should be changed for next time?").

Limits – Lay out **clear and fixed** limits, and remain resolute in applying them.

Feelings – People with the syndrome find it hard to phrase and express their feelings. Therefore, use questioning or checking to help him express himself ("I have the impression that it made you angry, is that how you feel?"). This will help you get authentic information from him.

Instill in him positive thoughts about himself – this a genuine gift that you give him. Confirm his **strengths**, which he believes he possesses ("I see that you're a positive, intelligent person and that you are capable of doing any job with the proper support").

Actions and their results – An issue that calls for attention as it is difficult for the adult with Asperger's (ASD) to perceive this intuitively. Rules and limitations are like the laws of nature. They must **be phrased clearly:** "If you do such and such….it will lead to better results."

Team Work – Help the worker feel good working in a team, **and help him understand**, as needed, "what is going on" in the team he belongs to.

Creating a joint base for discussion and mutual understanding in order to overcome situations of conflict will lead to **pleasant and fruitful** work relationships.

SUMMARY AND CONCLUSIONS

Integrating the concepts of occupational rehabilitation that focuses on the individual, and of supportive employment in a friendly and accepting workplace, enables the creation of optimal conditions for successful placement and upgrading the quality of life for adults with Asperger's (ASD).

* Inspired by the book by Bill Goodyear (2008), *Coaching People With Asperger's Syndrome*, London: Karnac Books.

I – SUITABLE EMPLOYMENT

CHAPTER 7: PREPARING FOR A SUCCESSFUL CAREER FOR ADULTS WITH ASPERGER'S (ASD)

INTRODUCTION

This chapter will discuss how to help prepare for a career, with emphasis on enhancing the self-esteem of each participant, based on his personal profile and needs. It is noteworthy that the search and internalization of information about themselves is of great importance for adults with Asperger's (ASD), before entering the workforce and in general. The most suitable employment is that which is based on the individual's strengths, and thus will minimize the disturbances his difficulties may cause, taking place in a work environment that is understanding, flexible, supportive and encouraging. This preliminary preparation can lead young high school graduates toward readiness for acquiring further education or a vocation. As to the adult group, even though most of them acquired an academic education, they have remained with difficulties in integrating into the workforce or persevering on the job and developing a career. Therefore they require preliminary training, both in the managerial and social aspects of their employment.

This chapter provides a response via workshops that will address the various issues related to working in an organized framework with other colleagues and under authority figures, in order to supply the adults with the syndrome with the tools they lack, suited to the individual potential abilities of each one. These workshops, however, represent only a small sample of the many venues for training and preparation toward successful employment. The facilitator will be expected to develop additional workshops that will meet the needs of his group and its members.

WORKSHOPS: PROVIDING TOOLS TO COPE WITH THE CHALLENGE OF EMPLOYMENT

SESSION 1 – LIFE SKILLS TO IMPROVE ADJUSTMENT TO THE JOB

INTRODUCTION

1. Getting acquainted through the facilitator's and the participants' self introduction.
2. Conditions for adjustment and integration at the workplace – a brief introduction presented by the facilitator.

Undoubtedly, skillful performance and talent at work receive their due respect, but this is not the case if one neglects his **personal grooming and hygiene**, which is **the basis** for all social skills (Grandin and Duffy, 2004).

These are the major points to focus on:

a. Personal grooming and how one dresses – invest in suitable clothing and see that it is clean. The type of clothing should be suited individually, with attention to the accepted dress code at the workplace and among your colleagues.
b. Physical cleanliness – daily attention – frequent change of clothing and **strict** use of deodorant. Whoever appears to be unkempt invites scorn and rejection.
c. Rigorous maintenance of a clean and orderly work environment – i.e., an uncluttered desk, without traces of coffee or unnecessary paper, etc. A neglected work area upsets others

and tarnishes the work milieu.

d.   Friendly integration into the workplace –also depends upon the efforts made by the employee to learn and internalize the accepted rules and adjust himself accordingly. He will thus also help his fellow workers to willingly be in his company and feel comfortable around him.

OUTLINE OF THE SESSION

The facilitator prepares copies of the above list of points and distributes them to all the group members. After a brief introduction in which he emphasizes the importance and significance of these points for adaptation to the workplace, he asks of each one to study the list and consider its contents. After three minutes, the group members are asked to give their reactions. The facilitator encourages each one to relate to the list and describe his attitude, feelings and difficulties. The purpose of the discussion is to lead the group to insights, awareness and internalization of these issues, as well as to deepen the fellowship between the members.

SESSION 2 – ACCEPTABLE AND UNACCEPTABLE BEHAVIORISMS AMONG COLLEAGUES

The facilitator begins by explaining the rationale and purpose of the meeting.

The accepted rules of behavior are: Keeping a distance of about half a meter when talking to colleagues. If you feel the need to express closeness or gratitude by touching your dialogue partner, it is customary to first ask his permission, such as: "Thank you for your help and support. Can I give you a hug, is that okay?" React accordingly. Exaggerated closeness to another person or even touching his things may stress him. The facilitator will invite each of the participants (to the center of the circle) and will demonstrate exaggerated closeness to him. It is important that the participants experience the feeling, to help them internalize the rule.

The next exercise is a demonstration of a short conversation at the proper distance. The group members will walk around the room and when encountering another person, they will stop for a two-minute conversation and try to maintain the right distance, and experience the feeling in this situation. Everyone should meet briefly with everyone else.

The last exercise of this session will address the issue of how to cope with the need to relax motoric activities, which appear strange to neurotypical colleagues and may cause them to distance themselves (Baker, 2005). For example: clapping hands, waving your arms, swaying your body, swinging your legs, etc. Baker suggests finding an alternative action that won't appear strange to others, such as: Holding something in your pocket that you can touch in order to relax. Each person should try to find what works best for him. After his opening remarks, the facilitator will lead a discussion on the subject, raising the issue of a person's need for a calming action. Additionally, he will encourage the participants to share with the group which motoric action calms them down, and will help raise suggested alternatives that do not draw the attention of others. The closing discussion will focus on the premise that everyone need not be alike. It is okay to be different, but important and desirable to moderate one's disparity with alternatives that please the eye.

SESSION 3 – ISSUES REGARDING THE CREATION OF A POSITIVE SELF-IMAGE (SELF-ADVOCACY)

To the facilitator – This session will focus on issues linked to the development and consolidation of a positive self-image of the adult with Asperger's (ASD) (at his workplace). Fast (2004) proposes some ideas that can contribute to the process of adjustment. She points out that the new employee is still in a learning stage, and needn't know everything. For people with Asperger's (ASD) the focus will be on acquiring the accepted behavior codes at the workplace, rules of human relations and acquiring social skills, all of which form the basis of this issue.

Success at the workplace for an employee with the syndrome does not depend only on his professional assets. His efforts to cause those around him to feel comfortable with him carry a lot of weight as well. During this time period, the major challenge is adjusting to the framework. In order to realize that, he must learn the organizational culture, the procedures and principles, and understand the rules by which things are done. It is important **to invest** effort in learning the organization's structure, its values, its key personnel, etc. One should become familiar with the personnel and their role, with the company's policies and both its formal and informal work procedures.

The approach of the program offered here suggests that during this trial period the employee with the syndrome be closely accompanied by a mentor who will coach him and also mediate between the employee and the staff he belongs to, in order to create understanding and insights from both sides. Emphasis will be placed on helping the new worker understand the system from all angles, on the one hand, and providing support for the staff, to help them understand and be tolerant and patient, on

322 | Benjamina Eran

the other hand. This coaching should be as intensive and as close as possible, for a period of four months, advisably once a week. Following that, in the spirit of this program, it is recommended to hold regular one-on-one follow-up meetings.

The facilitator begins the session with a discussion of the importance, during the first period at work, of creating a positive social image and explains the background (see the introduction to this session). The discussion is then summarized on an optimistic note: Even though the initial period of the first few months is difficult for workers with Asperger's (ASD), investing efforts in adjustment will bring relief further on. This, on condition that they learn to correct the social mistakes as early as possible, so that the criticisms and stigmas, if they have begun to form, do not take root among the colleagues.

STAGE A

Following the preliminary discussion, the group is divided into pairs. Each member of the pair plays a different role. Role A – The participant writes down how he sees himself making a positive impression or negative impression on his colleagues and superiors in the company. Role B – The participant writes down how he thinks the person in Role A can make a positive impression on his colleagues at work. After three minutes, each one reads to the other what he has written, they discuss it and clarify where they agree and where they disagree. (To **the facilitator:** It is important to prep the participants so that they accept their partner's feedback as help and not as an attack. Though they themselves are sensitive to criticism, yet they tend to give feedback to others in a coarse manner, not out of bad intent, but for lack of skills in tactful and pragmatic communication.)

STAGE B

The pairs change partners – all those who fulfilled Role A choose a partner who was in Role B, then continue working as in Stage A (after switching roles).

STAGE C

A group discussion (being flexible with the time), to enable the group to clear up any misunderstandings or disagreements that arose during the pairs' discussion, and to bring to closure whatever issues remained unresolved.

SESSION 4 – BEHAVIOR CODES AT THE WORKPLACE

This session will be more open in comparison to the other sessions. Its **first** part will deal with "taking the group's temperature," i.e., each participant will relate what he has learned about himself, what he still finds difficult to do and how he feels about it. If the group members express themselves in brief and everyone speaks in turn, thus ending the round quickly, the remaining time can be devoted to discussing behavior codes at the workplace and the meaning of authoritarian relationships vs. relationships between equals, etc.

Fast (2004) suggests that the new worker observe his colleagues, follow the dynamics between them and study their habits. For example, do they work behind closed doors? What do they talk about? How do they dress? How do they behave at staff meetings? What is the attitude toward coming late or absence from meetings? What takes place at informal meetings? What are the various channels of communication? Are electronic systems networking the offices or is it personal communication? How do the executives communicate with their subordinates?

It is advisable to encourage the participants to interview friends, family, etc., in order to learn from them about the norms and regulations at their places of work.

SESSION 5 – ORGANIZATIONAL SKILLS REQUIRED FOR SUCCESS ON THE JOB

During the fifth session, emphasis will be placed on the rules of behavior that can be learned. The focus will be on mandatory organizational skills for success at work. The various issues are:

1. Planning long-term objectives.
2. Defining goals.
3. A time schedule for completing the tasks.
4. A daily time schedule.
5. The ways of implementation.
6. Priorities.
7. Making decisions.
8. Problem-solving.

The facilitator describes a project that is about to begin at an imaginary workplace, in which the group participants are **hypothetically** the employees, and the manager has instructed each one of them to plan this project. The facilitator will ask of each member to write down one example for each of the above issues. The facilitator has to prepare the name of the project and the nature of the company in which the project is implemented, suited to the participants' level and their occupation or education. The project should be linked to a familiar topic.

Alternatively, a project can be prepared for each participant individually that is suited to his professional or occupational designation. Each of the participants will be asked to write a program for his project, addressing the first five issues noted above. The issues relating to priorities, decision-making and problem-solving (items 6-8) will be clarified by the entire group, after each participant has read the first five items. The facilitator will lead the discussion and will teach these issues in a practical manner, while relating to the questions raised in the group discussion.

The concluding discussion will focus on **the conclusions** of each of the participants as to what he has learned and internalized about himself and the others.

I – SUITABLE EMPLOYMENT
CHAPTER 8: FACING SUCCESS IN YOUR CAREER

A SUMMARIZING DISCUSSION

Grandin and Duffy (2004) claim that in order to succeed on the job, helpful intervention is required for people with Asperger's (ASD) through every transitional stage into a life of employment.

In this regard, it is worth emphasizing the significance of structured and well-organized preparation within the framework of a consistent and professional rehabilitation program, and its impact on one's success in his career.

LIFE SKILLS – Life skills begin with the most basic tasks, such as being well-groomed and looking after the immediate physical environment (order and cleanliness). Grandin relates how her supervisor at work assigned his secretary to take her shopping for clothes, and asked her to use deodorant. Though at that moment she didn't appreciate his directness, she learned later on that he had done her a huge favor.

ORGANIZATIONAL SKILLS – These have a direct impact on how the adult with the syndrome conducts himself at work at all levels, from planning and up to implementing. These skills influence his basic conduct, such as: Arriving to work on time, adjusting a schedule to an overload of tasks by prioritizing, having a clear and orderly definition of goals, objectives and tasks, and managing financial matters. Additionally, these include personal skills, such as managing a detailed daily work schedule, ascertaining to implement and time the program, and attendance and participation in staff missions.

Moreover, the value of the computer and its efficient use, along with the internet, should not be overlooked for preparing presentations, for ongoing communication, locating data, etc.

SOCIAL SKILLS – Grandin and Duffy (2004) maintain that employment is largely a social activity and therefore it is important that a person with Asperger's (ASD) learn how to work **with others**. He must be familiar with his own limitations, to ensure that he can avoid problematic situations or know how to correct mistakes. Notwithstanding, it is important to continue training in order to develop social skills.

Social skills also include the ability to take part in a conversation and form a connection with supportive colleagues. This is a significant factor in helping workers with Asperger's (ASD) navigate their way wisely within the organization. It is also a source of help in understanding the social rules and norms.

This category also includes training toward assertiveness and an essential understanding of authority relationships. Assertiveness helps adults with Asperger's (ASD) self-advocate and maintain ties with their colleagues from an established stand, without callousness or anger. This kind of communication helps express confidently and in a balanced way the strengths and compatibilities of the adult with Asperger's (ASD), and his ability to contribute to his workplace. In this manner, a healthy infrastructure is created for developing an open, honest communication between the staff workers and enables an open channel for a friendly, supportive relationship from the supervisors as well.

Integrity also strengthens the colleagues and supervisors' trust in the new employee with Asperger's (ASD). They appreciate his honesty and learn that he can be trusted. This promotes cooperation between the parties and further deepens their understanding of his 'strange' behaviorisms. Instead of whispering behind his back or being critical toward him, the staff will increasingly want to help him. With mutual trust, the employee will receive and internalize their suggestions more easily. This ties in with the training in assertiveness that he acquired during his pre-employment training period, and with the self-advocacy skills he developed, along with his self-confidence, which increased during the rehabilitation process. This is a process of developing self-awareness, of recognizing one's talents, cognitive abilities, fields of interest and successes that are all part of a positive self-definition. It also includes understanding the problematic areas he must cope with. When his relationship with his fellow worker is supportive and there is an open dialogue between them, communication increases that benefits both him and the organization.

One of the cases presented by Fast (2004) in her book is an informative description of the conditions needed to facilitate a thriving career for the adult with Asperger's (ASD) and, contrarily, what are the harmful effects of their absence:

Fast was a bookworm and was outstanding in her humanities studies. As a child, she was considered strange, despite her strong desire to fit in socially. She was successful at work because of her high work ethic, her great productivity and her drive to satisfy others. Her supervisor was a nice person, and her colleagues showed interest in her knowledge. All this took place in her country of origin.

She then moved to a new place, where she studied for an advanced degree, was accepted for a job on campus and was quickly promoted, because she succeeded in developing interesting projects and proposals for greater efficiency. Additionally, at the same time, she was diagnosed with Asperger's (ASD). Her work environment was characterized by serious, devoted workers and a thoroughgoing, logical supervisor who greatly appreciated her hard work and commitment. Most of her colleagues showed tolerance of what was different about her, and they weren't very competitive. Even though everyone noticed that she talks to herself, they greatly admired her for her persistent work, her commitment and desire to help, and her suggestions for improvement. Under these conditions, Fast was able to turn her strengths to an advantage and minimize her weaknesses.

She invested great effort in turning her disadvantages into advantages, by developing skills that she could apply toward this goal. She improved her communication and social skills, and found a way of overcoming her difficulty in identifying faces. She graduated with honors and was hired to work in another university. In her new environment, she was treated coldly, others took over her desk and her phone, and hid from her the entry code into the computer. These harassments increased over time. She didn't quit and continued trying as best she could to provide the finest service, but her supervisor continued thwarting her. She learned that in her department it was important to belong to a certain group of workers and their supervisor, and to know how to navigate herself within the departmental politics. However, her social communication skills were insufficient to meet the task.

This story illustrates the critical elements that impact on the success or failure of a person coping with Asperger's (ASD). Fast (2004) represents those adults with the syndrome who enter the

330 | Benjamina Eran

workforce with great motivation and goodwill. For lack of an organized rehabilitation program, most of them are forced to walk down this unfamiliar, enigmatic path alone.

Not all of them have the stamina, willpower and ambition to contribute to and satisfy the organization, as Fast did. Yet this is not sufficient. Like in most aspects of life, 'it takes two to tango'. When she found a partner who adjusted himself to her and provided work conditions that were considerate, accepting and encouraging, she flowered and excelled.

Apparently, the question that arises is: How is this connected to Asperger's (ASD)? The same thing can happen to others as well. The answer is rather complex: There is no doubt that the conditions in Fast's last employment would be unbearable for any worker. However, any non-supportive system, even if it isn't antagonistic as the one she experienced, is assumedly impossible for people with Asperger's (ASD), because the skills required to deal with intra-organizational politics are lacking. They have a hard time understanding sophisticated language, such as humor, metaphors and cynical statements. They do not easily understand non-verbal communication such as body language, gestures, etc. They are also limited in their ability to read the social map and understand interpersonal dynamics.

From this data, it is understandable how complex is the difficulty that prevents people with Asperger's (ASD) to successfully belong to a social framework, even when it is not thwarting or antagonistic.

The solution lies in a **comprehensive** rehabilitation framework that will provide the proper solutions to these problems. There is widespread agreement among many who have delved into the syndrome's enigmas that it is possible to improve to some degree the skills that are lacking, in accordance with the individual potential of each person. Assuming that the rehabilitation programs will include a variety of workshops on training, practice and advancement in all the problematic areas, there is room to believe that upgrading the abilities and skills of the participants will enable them to integrate into an accepting and supportive work framework.

The optimal investment in imbuing these skills should be significantly helpful to the rehabilitant adult with Asperger's (ASD) in consolidating employment goals in a **logical** way, in entering the workforce at a good level of **preparedness** and in achieving successful **absorption**.

II – BEING IN A COUPLE RELATIONSHIP
WITH ASPERGER'S (ASD)

CHAPTER 1: BEING IN A COUPLE RELATIONSHIP WITH ASPERGER'S (ASD) – HOW IS IT POSSIBLE?

INTRODUCTION TO THE FACILITATORS

It is often said that adults with Asperger's (ASD) are not capable of intimate relationships (Lovett 2005). Such an approach ends any hope for family life and integration into a close and stable relationship. Therefore, every consideration should be given to any sustainable possibility for improving the quality of life of these adults and supporting every couple that pursues such a relationship.

Every couple is a unique human entity and is entitled to an acceptance and understanding of the ways of adjustment suitable to them.

Couples who have succeeded in maintaining a long-term family relationship teach us that a strong will and a loving commitment are the building blocks for establishing a stable couple relationship throughout life.

Hendrickx et al (2007) in their book, *Asperger – A Love Story*, take us along the path of their life journey, both separately and together, toward a satisfying couple relationship. Each of the two claims that **communication** is the most essential key for establishing and maintaining family life and experiencing a close and stable relationship. Though Asperger's (ASD) is a syndrome marked by difficulties in the interpersonal and social spheres, nonetheless we –the therapists, rehabilitators and mentors – must weigh **every opportunity** that may **improve** the quality of life of these adults. Each one of them is an individual, and every couple has its own unique dynamics, for 'wondrous are the ways of mankind'.

The obvious stand in this regard is: If we don't try, how will we know? Research on couples with Asperger's (ASD) and thera-peutic approaches are still in the very early stages, and do not justify precluding any possibilities. Books written by couples who succeeded in maintaining a long-term family framework open a window for those with the syndrome, and for professionals as well, and prove that a strong will and loving commitment can bring about remarkable results. The key phrase in this regard is provided by Stanford (2006): "I fervently believe that there are ways to help build a lifelong relationship with a mate who has Asperger's (ASD). I believe that in order to find such solutions, an exceptional level of devotion is required."

A couple with Asperger's (ASD) finds it hard to understand and internalize accepted rules and gestures and communicate with others beyond the clear meaning of the spoken word, whereas the neurotypical partner in a couple relationship can create empathy and understand his or her mate (Stanford, 2006).

Hendrickx et al (2007) in their book, *Asperger Syndrome – A Love Story*, take us step by step down the paths of their lives, along which they strode alone and together on their way to a sat-isfying relationship. Their story illustrates what Nietzsche once said: "He who has what to live for can bear any path." Each one in this couple states that **communication** is the essential key, through which one can listen and develop mutual acceptance.

Sara, the neurotyical partner of this couple, learned how to understand and communicate in "Asperger-ese," as if it were her second language, and was easily able to translate the language of her thoughts. It found expression in bridging between the different ways of perception and adjustment in an equal acceptance of each other's ways, as well as giving each other living space that allows each one to be himself and to learn to accept himself. The concluding sentence of the partner with Asperger's (ASD) testifies to the outcome of the mental efforts the couple invested in their consistency and persistence. He states that his wife's acceptance of Asperger's (ASD) changed his life. Prior to that he was isolated and felt guilty. Today, **he has a life.**

In the introduction to the book by the couple, Gisela and Christopher Slater-Walker (2002), they assert that adults with the syndrome are capable of developing a successful relationship with a partner. They state that parents and clinicians may have doubts as to that, and therefore it is essential to become familiar with some key factors regarding adults with Asperger's (ASD) and their mates. A partner in a couple relationship can acquire skills for functioning within a relationship, by applying his cognitive skills more than his intuition. The primary condition is that the couple has **motivation, as well as training and escorting,** in everything related to affection and relations. Those diagnosed with the syndrome bring into a couple relationship valuable traits, such as trustworthiness, integrity, honesty, etc. Nonetheless, mental effort is required to maintain the relationship with one's mate. The couple relationship presents an ongoing challenge, and in order to establish it, mental investment is needed throughout the long-term process of mutual adjustment. In couple relationships in general, and with Asperger's (ASD) in particular, the question of nurturing intimate emotional relations, together with **reciprocal** dependency, is a far greater challenge. The core difficulties of the syndrome, i.e., the difficulty in understanding the thoughts and feelings of others, together with a lack of flexibility, makes it hard to create closeness, emotional intimacy and mutual support, which are so essential in a couple relationship (Lovett,2005). In contrast, understanding and accepting the syndrome by both partners is an important key toward accepting their being different and toward their success as a couple. Lovett raises the **conjecture** that the intimacy between two partners in a couple relationship, both of whom have Asperger's (ASD), will lead to a mutual understanding between them. A different conjecture is no less relevant: It points to the fact that because of the special difficulties of the partner with Asperger's (ASD), it is essential that his mate demonstrate openness and flexibility in the relationship, and be able to show acceptance and empathy, perseverance, patience and open-mindedness. It is important that one of the partners be capable of holding and preserving this shared unit while maintaining respect for his partner's special needs.

II - BEING IN A COUPLE RELATIONSHIP
WITH ASPERGER'S (ASD)

CHAPTER 2: SOCIAL INTELLIGENCE -
THE BASIS FOR SUCCESS IN FRIENDSHIPS AND IN
COUPLE RELATIONSHIPS

Social intelligence is expressed via the capacity to adjust to people and to social situations. In the workshops for social life skills, we train adults with Asperger's (ASD) whose inherent social abilities are lacking, therefore they need structured and focused training in this area. The aim of the workshops is to expand and reinforce the various social skills and equip the adults with the capability of coping in interpersonal relations, which will improve their adjustment and success in the different areas of life, such as career, society, couple relationships and family.

In his book, *Social Intelligence*, Albrecht (2010) defines, describes and details the behaviorisms that are characteristic of efficient interpersonal abilities, as opposed to obstructive behaviorisms.

Social intelligence - An integration between a basic understanding of people and the skills that enable successful interaction. This includes the ability to minimize confrontations and create a cooperative environment, and apply skills that go beyond accepted politeness.

Albrecht suggests the phrase **effective human approach** as a concept for understanding situations and social contexts. In the process of neurotypical development, this trait is acquired via observation and self learning. **Nurturing behaviorisms** are usually acquired in this manner, and they encourage one's partner to feel that he is capable, loved, accepted and self-assured. In contrast, there are some behavioral manifestations that thwart the ability to conduct sound social integration.

In relating to **skills in interpersonal relationships,** Albrecht notes the following traits:

1. **Social radar** – Enables to read the emotional state of another person.
2. **Presence** – An assemblage of signs that can be integrated and used to assess one's impression and evaluation of others. This includes a person's outer appearance and behavioral traits.
3. **Genuineness** – Integrity, openness, ethics, trust.
4. **Clarity in communication** – The ability to explain and express oneself in an easily understood manner (talking only as necessary, being skilled in active listening, saying the right thing at the right time and explaining one's position convincingly).
5. **Empathy** – An emotional connection by understanding the other, as a basis for cooperation.
6. Being able to **accept feedback from others**.
7. Being able to **feel and decipher others' reactions** to social stress, confrontation, uncertainty, and to respond intuitively in real time.
8. Understanding **the social context**- This creates meaningful communication and influences the behavior of those involved. Different connections will bestow a different meaning to the social context, and that is why people who are self-centered frequently miss the relevance of the connections and respond **erroneously**. Typical contexts are: The

physical environment, the participants' behavior patterns and emotional nuances, as well as the level of understanding, linguistic habits, social codes, behavior norms, the quality of the relationships, cultural differences and relationships of authority or equality. Being self-centered is expressed in **the absence** of empathy and genuineness.

9. **Semantic deficiencies** – According to Albrecht (2010), these include: Being opinionated, dogmatic, generalizing, tagging and being ironic. In contrast, using metaphors is a tool to help understand intentions and meanings beyond the spoken words, on condition that they are suitable to the dialogue partner's thought flexibility. For example: 'to get into your head' cannot be interpreted literally. The meaning is to learn what motivates a person and what makes him react as he does. Albrecht clarifies those concepts that describe the abilities and deficiencies in social functioning. These are relevant to our topic, as they define social abilities on the one hand, and limited, hindering abilities on the other hand. Both of these can be used to enrich the 'tool kit' in the workshops for developing social skills and **reciprocal and couple relationships.**

II – BEING IN A COUPLE RELATIONSHIP WITH ASPERGER'S (ASD)
CHAPTER 3: THE ELUSIVE EXPERIENCE AND THE NEUROTYPICAL CULTURE

INTRODUCTION

In his paper, "Bridging the Gaps: A Look at Autism from the Inside," Sinclair (at www.sinclair.org) describes his personal experiences, presenting them and their significance. Following is an extract of his thoughts and conclusions:

"A look from the Inside"

1. Usually, I understand when I don't understand something, and can identify the gaps between what I actually don't understand to what others assume it is that I understand.
2. The source of autism is in the neurological variance with all its diverse consequences.
3. The difficulty lies in identifying and processing stimuli to introduce order into the chaos.
4. The most recurrent factor is the gap between what is expected to be taught and what is assumedly already understood.
5. My questions are mostly ignored or are treated with distrust.
6. I am punished because of my intelligence, because I am considered "smart enough" to understand things on my own (the Elusive syndrome).
7. I couldn't find employment, because others assumed that I understand what is expected of me, and I know how to carry through, yet I fail intentionally or out of hostility.

8. I had a friend who lacked any psychological training, yet understood some of my characteristics and guided me in several ways, such as: Never assume **anything**, that is, **ask** instead of **guessing**.

9. Those around me always assumed that if my emotions are not **visible**, it is not possible that I am capable of **feeling** them. This is a terrible mistake made by neurotypical people in their ability to understand another person's viewpoint.

10. I met someone who spoke a lot about her feelings, who identified the concept that represented the feeling and where she felt it. She would clarify for me whatever I asked. I understood that it is possible to use words to describe personal experiences, and I have continued using this tool.

11. Unfounded assumptions regarding another person's feelings create barriers to mutual understanding and harm a relationship (deficient communication).

12. Regardless of my intellect, my appearance remains strange, and people doubt my ability to reach reasonable conclusions, only because I didn't reach more 'appropriate' decisions.

13. I am blamed for being purposely insensitive, **for how can anyone comprehend that someone doesn't understand?**

14. Neurotypical people usually tend to minimize my difficulties and deny my abilities.

15. I cannot always follow what is taking place around me, but I am never disconnected from my internal being. Even when I am incapable of focusing, I still have my self, but I am not apathetic to my surroundings.

Additional Gaps Related to Interpersonal Functioning

1. The accepted attitude is that the way I relate to others is different from the norm, due to indifference or a negative attitude toward them.

2. The answer to that is that autistic people usually lack an awareness of social cues, therefore they also have a limited capacity to decipher social and environmental situations.

3. This is a kind of 'hidden blindness' which causes the autist not to discern facial expressions, and when he does discern them, he finds it hard to understand their meaning or how to deal with it. When people say it is out of indifference, it is insulting and despairing.

4. When a relationship is formed by choice, it is a special experience, and the partner in this relationship is the most important thing in the world for the other one with Asperger's (ASD).

5. In the social milieu, what is prominent is the difficulty in following all that is happening at once, and we need help in getting explanations.

6. Being a high-functioning autist does not mean being non-human. On the contrary – we have the ability to **learn** how to form relationships.

Sinclair ends his paper on a personal (though representative) note: "Don't try to change me to fit your world. Form contact with me in my world, work together with me in order to build bridges."

342 | Benjamina Eran

II – BEING IN A COUPLE RELATIONSHIP WITH ASPERGER'S (ASD)

CHAPTER 4: COPING WITH THE ISSUE OF EMOTIONS

Williams (1996) addresses the confusing issue for autists of understanding emotions. She clarifies the connection between physical reactions to emotional reactions, and thus is able to help everyone involved (parents, teachers, clinicians, adults with Asperger's (ASD), as well as their partners and friends).

Her writing is based on understanding how the brain functions for those diagnosed on the autistic spectrum. She points out two types: The first is manifested by a lack of understanding feedback – in which case there is no emotional stimulation. The second type is a lack of translating physical feedback into emotional significance. The neurotypical adult expects his dialogue partner to recognize a range of emotions and cannot understand why he isn't connecting.

Williams (1996) points out two additional mechanisms that exist at the sensory level: The first is linked to **increased** sensory sensitivity, which can also influence the emotional level (caution = dread; dissatisfaction = frustration; sadness = depression). Such experiences may be overwhelming and raise the need for caution from social involvement. The second mechanism – derives from receiving constructive feedback that is interpreted as judgmental criticism. This type of experience brings about emotional confusion and may turn into an experience of rejection, arousing the hurt party's need to avoid social exposure.

The writer testifies about herself that she fights her autism, because she wants to live her life and create deep and long-term relationships.

She concludes with an encouraging appeal: "Be proud of who you are... it is your business to cope with it...."

This paper opens a window for people with the syndrome, and to the interpersonal and neurotypical world – to the inner and emotional world of the autists. Additionally, she opens a window for parents - to their children, for caregivers – to their patients, between friends and, no less important - **to couples and to whoever is engaged in a long-term relationship.**

II – BEING IN A COUPLE RELATIONSHIP WITH ASPERGER'S (ASD)

CHAPTER 5: THE FACTORS THAT PRESERVE THE "TOGETHERNESS" OF A COUPLE

Joselson (1996) throws light on those factors that influence the "togetherness" of a couple and motivate them, despite their individual differences:

BELONGING

This is a significant factor contributing to physical health, longevity, a meaningful social life, growth and development, setting boundaries and developing the self **as a result of integrating with others.**

In the adult's life, **emotional support** means helping someone else, to avoid a crisis or come out of one. Support is the basis for the experience upon which a shared life is built.

We are supported by networks of meaningfulness that comfort us in that they provide us with a sense of, belonging and **hope.**

ATTACHMENT

Attachment is a state in which we remain close to someone, and we need to know that he is close and accessible and that it will continue into the future, otherwise there is nothing to depend on and one's security isn't guaranteed. Attachment is the feeling of **emotional belonging.**

However, some people experience attachment as a prison of

sorts. They perceive it as undermining their independence, and apparently there are personal differences between the level of attachment or degree of autonomy that each person is in need of.

EYE CONTACT

A loving glance is a glance of appreciation, of our being special and important to others, which gives us a sense of meaning in relation to the world. We need the feeling that we are wanted in the world in which we live. **Our being significant** to another person justifies our existence and empowers our feeling that indeed we are important in the eyes of someone who loves us for who we are.

RECIPROCITY

Reciprocity is a joint creation that exists with the help of shared mental situations. It develops jointly between people, where each one **contributes and takes part**. Therefore, within reciprocity, **"us"** is of principal importance.

THE SEARCH FOR RECIPROCITY

The search for reciprocity illuminates those aspects of the personal experience that can be shared with others. Reciprocity exists between friends, in ongoing relationships and in couple relationships. With reciprocity, the pleasure from the experience itself is very important. Reciprocity is the expression of the basic social nature of human beings.

The experience of **together**, of **us**, is reinforced by reciprocity and the pleasure nurtures the desire to continue the connection that has been created.

DEVOTION AND CARING ABOUT OTHERS

This type of connection requires several forms of empathy. Initially, one must discover what the partner **needs and is capable** of receiving. Additionally, we must feel empathy for his anxiety, and as a result of that, a desire to quieten him. The outcome will be that we give him strength, while at the same time we will be able **to express** ourselves and **receive** in return emotional warmth directed at us.

In order to express **empathy**, one needs to be emotionally mature.

In order to feel what others are experiencing, there is a need for employing awareness and empathy. Since every person has personal experiences and conflicts, self-awareness will help us recognize that it isn't always possible to understand the other person emotionally. Empathy is the basis of the desire to understand, to help, protect, encourage and calm down another person.

Devotion is a central factor in belonging, and presents a substantial challenge.

GENDER DIFFERENCES AND BELONGING

Belonging and connecting are important to both men and women. Mutual commitment is the empowering force enabling us to persevere in our efforts for a long-term and healthy relationship.

THE DIFFERENCE BETWEEN GENDERS is an encumbrance on the couple relationship. Nonetheless, it is a positive force toward the **mutual effort** of the couple **to deepen the understanding** and closeness between them in order to **cultivate a healthy relationship**.

II – BEING IN A COUPLE RELATIONSHIP WITH ASPERGER'S (ASD)

CHAPTER 6: THOUGHTS ON LOVE AND INTIMACY

LOVE/Yoram Taharlev [originally in Hebrew]
Love is a very vague feeling
At times it's a touch, at times it is speaking,
At times it's just a glance, at times a fleeting thought,
At times it's being distant, and at times being near,
But if in your heart you feel a kind of clicking,
Be not alarmed, it will do no harm.
A racing heart, irregular breathing,
It's not an illness, it is simply love.

Every person has his own personal "menu" of his need for love. The quality of love changes, as it contains multiple dimensions.

A sense of failure within a relationship between kindred of the first degree, at times stems from the fantasy that one person can provide all the needs of his partner. When someone says "I love," he means that someone or something is very significant to him, or that the object of his love arouses a strong positive response in him.

Love is communicating and connecting with the loved one. It is based on the assumption that he is special and unique.

Most of us experience different forms of love from early childhood, within our immediate family and with other people close to us. Such relationships sustain a variety of needs.

Love is the **longing** of one person for another, the attraction to **a connection,** to a relationship of **reciprocity** and joint experiences. It contains **gratitude** for the understanding, acceptance and security received, and the answer to the **emotional** need to "**be at home.**"

Our love is offered also to those who strengthen us, who serve as a mirror for us, who make us feel that they complete us, that with them we can share the ups and downs of life.

During the process of connecting and growing within a couple relationship, we gradually **discover our selves**. We experience changing relationships and learn to adjust. We grow closer to others, we progress in **building the "us,"** while at the same time we respect **the uniqueness of each other.**

Not being loved – means that we are not significant or important, which invites pain.

People live with their fantasy of love, on the one hand, and with their real experiences, on the other hand, and they must face these gaps.

In conclusion, within the framework of **couple relationships,** both **the internal and external, the self and the other,** co-exist - as do **nearness and distance, fantasy and reality**, rationality and irrationality, **the conscious and the unconscious.** In other words, a long-term relationship is a complex relationship that changes and develops over time and those within the relationship need to possess openness, tolerance, patience **and the commitment to continue to invest** in it and nurture it.

II – BEING IN A COUPLE RELATIONSHIP WITH ASPERGER'S (ASD)

CHAPTER 7: ASPERGER'S (ASD) – A LOVE STORY

The Hendrickx couple (2007) relates in their book how the beginning of their relationship was marked by chaos and confusion and that their relationship came to a harsh and painful end. However, despite it all and rather because of this experience, they succeeded in building a more satisfying relationship and they learned to recognize that they are happier together than apart. Naturally, each one is different from the other, therefore each couple copes with the difficulties of understanding one another. However, when one member of the couple is diagnosed with Asperger's (ASD), they must bridge over an especially great gap, with added hardships and challenges more so than a neurotypical couple.

This couple recounts their shared adjustment process, and concludes that the key is **communication,** along with the readiness, constancy and persistence to cope together. They report that they learned that there is no right or wrong, and that it is possible to **accept, compromise and enjoy what there is.**

Everything said so far is characteristic of any couple, but in reality, this isn't the case. The woman in the Hendrickx partnership attests about herself, that she learned **to translate** the words and behavior of her partner with the syndrome into her own language of thought. In this way, she helped her partner to better understand both the verbal and non-verbal neurotypical communication. She learned by experience that investing effort and diligence can have significant impact in the long run. According to her, the conclusion is that it is best to **lay aside** negative energies from the shared past **and communicate with positive energies**. Additionally, it is recommended to treat your partner with appreciation and respect **for what he is** and who he is, and for love.

In conclusion, this couple's experience testifies to the fact that there are a number of principles that help preserve a relationship, and they are: Unconditional love, open, flowing communication, effort, perseverance and investment. All of this applies to neuro-typical couples as well, for each partner in a couple relationship brings to the connection between the two his own perceptions, values, habits and unique personality. Therefore, **a conflict** is an opportunity to **reinforce the relationship**, through sympathetic communication, and accepting the differences of opinion as **an opportunity** to deepen one's familiarity with the perceptions, habits and desires that are both similar and different. Thus, a couple relationship can develop that is based on openness, understanding and mutual acceptance.

II – BEING IN A COUPLE RELATIONSHIP WITH ASPERGER'S (ASD)

CHAPTER 8: ASPERGER'S (ASD) AND LONG-TERM RELATIONSHIPS

Stanford (2006), in her book about the relationship of a couple where the man had Asperger's (ASD) and the woman was neuro-typical, suggests **optimism** as an empowering tool that provides the strength to look to the future positively, helps solve problems and **supports the survival** of the relationship. She refers to optimism that **is based on reality, and building a bridge** over the gaps **from the start** of the couple relationship.

Additionally, she points to factors that impact on the development of interpersonal skills for adults with Asperger's (ASD), and that aggravate the couple's communication. Here are some examples:

a. Failure in creating relationships of friendship, suited to the developmental age.

b. A history of rejection, provocations and harassments that left emotional scars.

c. Memories of past failures in attempts to connect with others.

d. The absence of the ability to identify cues that give a warning of entering into undesirable situations, and how to get out of them.

e. Entering into a couple relationship with no experience in long-term relationships.

f.   The neurotypical partner expects a sharing of experiences and perceptions, in a relationship marked by **mutual** gentleness, warmth and concern. He copes with **a constant** search for the most appropriate way to reinforce and deepen the couple relationship.

Following is a sample of the hardships and challenges in everyday life:

1.   A lack of spontaneity of the partner with Asperger's (ASD) in seeking out shared pleasures (social, romantic and intimate).
2.   A lack of initiative and sharing.
3.   A reduction in emotional and social reciprocity.
4.   Difficulty in understanding and containing the sophisticated complexity of long-term reciprocal relationships.
5.   Difficulty in behaving according to the rules and norms in their different contexts.
6.   Employing harsh and tactless "truths," i.e., speaking the truth at any price, **without understanding its consequences.**

When the couple shares a basic connection of love, commitment and faith in a long-term process of honest communication, they will progress toward an optimistic future based on reality. It is recommended to be helped by professional support and guidance, as needed.

II – BEING IN A COUPLE RELATIONSHIP WITH ASPERGER'S (ASD)
CHAPTER 9: BREAKING THE GLASS CEILING OF LONELINESS

Rest assured, seek with all your might and you shall find.

Dawn Prince-Hughes (2006) in her autobiographical book, *Songs of the Gorilla Nation,* sums up what she has learned and **implemented** from her caring for gorillas, during which time she developed meaningful communication and significant ties with them. Changes that she experienced vis-a-vis **human beings** brought her to a point that she "couldn't have dreamed of" before, including communicating her skills to others, and knowing when it is time to end a conversation. She found interest in **other people** and adopted **more moderate** opinions. She is careful to maintain **eye contact**, to read **emotions** of others and react in a way that will help them feel good. The more she applied these skills, the easier and more natural they became for her, and with time she applied these skills to **express appreciation** toward others, especially those she likes.

She still feels tense in public places, especially when she thinks people are looking at her. The human face remains a **challenge** for her, therefore she learned to pretend that she recognizes her acquaintances. The **clamor** in the streets is still hard for her. She describes how she **copes** with anxieties: She wears the same clothes again and again, she sleeps in these clothes, compulsively clears her throat in social situations, and leaves her house an hour earlier to reach a **new place**. In addition, she needs **to clarify** with her close friends **if she understood** the meaning of what was said at an event.

Living with her female **partner** has enabled her to learn and to trust, to overcome her fear of **change** and to believe that **flexibility** is important in all aspects of interpersonal life. She has learned **to let go of her need to control** and to pass on **responsibility** to others.

"At one time, I'd get stuck in one emotion and couldn't get out of it," Dawn confesses, and relates how she learned that **emotions pass**. In the past, she was afraid of disagreements or **anger**, and today she understands that it is possible to put it behind you with **a positive ending.** Her life partner has calmed her down and has taught her **to think of what can happen** later on, and try to accept things out of an understanding of what is happening **beyond the words**. She has learned **to take responsibility**, as well as support and protect those who are important to her.

Dawn sums it up by saying that she has learned to distinguish between what can be changed and what **cannot** be changed. Her words indicate that she has acquired a trustful compass that directs her how to conduct herself.

TRAITS AND DIFFICULTIES THAT TYPIFY ADULTS WITH ASPERGER'S (ASD)

Dawn Prince-Hughes describes the suffering of those people found on the autistic spectrum, and in her unique way she expresses their pain, with harsh words: Neurotypical people don't understand them, the way society treats them is **absurd**, they are perceived as **caricatures**. Society's **prejudices** lead to their exclusion, and they are **left behind.**

Dawn learned that these adults build their own culture, yet they "yearn to have others confirm their attempts and relate to them."

However, since her book was published, there has been an improvement in the position of research work and professional therapy methods. This change has also had a gradual impact on the attitude of the neurotypical society, and a window has been opened toward understanding and acceptance. However, this does not solve the anger and frustration, the anxiety and depression that result from failure and rejection.

Success in friendship and companionship **validates** our existential feeling and is crucial for emotional wellness and personal growth. Dawn relates in detail how her years at school left their scars on her, from the harassments from other children and the school's imperviousness. She also speaks of the tics, the special **sensitivities**, her **suspiciousness** toward authority and her **abstention** from social ties. In addition to all that, her **compulsiveness** was blatant in her manner of dress and strange manner of speech. This entire "package" generated in her childhood reactions of ostracism and painful aggression (she was beaten, kicked, spat at and called derogatory names).

Dawn points out that she grew up in an eccentric working-class family, of the type that were distrustful of psychologists. In her **extended** family, many adults were found to have autism of various degrees. When she was informed of the professional diagnosis of herself, she tried to reject it, recalling the many **stereotypes** that her environment holds to be true ("Aspergers don't have feelings, they don't have friends, or mates, they can't relate to others"). She lost her serenity, which led to a progressively

356 | B<small>ENJAMINA</small> E<small>RAN</small>

deep emotional **crisis**. Turning to **professional help** provided Dawn with the ability to embark on a process of acceptance, during which she would explain in her lectures that every person with Asperger's (ASD) knows he is different, but suffers from not knowing **why**, therefore it is safe to assume that his behavior won't change. She encouraged parents to seek out diagnosis and professional help.

Dawn began looking for ways that would help her reach a balance, and discovered anti-depressants and drugs for OCD (Obsessive-Compulsive Disorder). She took up relaxing activities and joined a group of "Academicians on the Autistic Spectrum." From discussions held in the group, she observed which of her behaviorisms originated from autistic factors and what was strange about her beyond that.

Her activities for **self-help** balanced and strengthened her endurance and persistence and **propelled her forward**. It began with **lectures** and meetings with relevant audiences, then continued with her **doctoral studies**, followed by **academic teaching** and planning a family with her **life partner** who gave birth to a **baby boy**. Dawn then discovered her **motherly** feelings for the first time, and burst out crying from joy with the baby's birth. In her own words, "These discoveries and my acceptance of them helped me **to better carry out human interaction**."

II – BEING IN A COUPLE RELATIONSHIP WITH ASPERGER'S (ASD)

CHAPTER 10: WAYS TO IMPROVE THE QUALITY OF LIFE FOR COUPLES WITH ASPERGER'S (ASD)

THE FOLLOWING IS A TWO-YEAR PROGRAM THAT IN-CLUDES A NUMBER OF EXPERIENCES:

THE ORGANIZATIONAL FRAMEWORK:

a. The program is targeted at candidates that have experience in a couple relationship, with or without joint habitation.

b. The candidates who are accepted have to complete the workshop for developing social life skills (See Part III in this book).

c. All the couples must commit to complete the entire program.

d. Each couple will undergo an intake interview of at least one hour, to consolidate their suitability.

e. It is desirable and **recommended** that the program be carried out by a pair of facilitators from both genders.

f. This is a program aimed exclusively for couples and **is not** suitable for individuals.

g. Every group session will last 120 minutes.

THE FIRST YEAR

The workshop for developing social life skills will meet once a week, for eight months, and will consist of 36 weekly sessions (additional assignments will be given that will include both individual and group tasks between sessions).

THE SECOND YEAR

Following a two-month break, the group will reconvene to continue the program within the framework of the **workshop** for improving the quality of life in couple relationships. The break will enable the couples to accumulate shared experiences and apply the tools they acquired in the previous workshop. The facilitators will provide the participants with a list of activities.

1. The workshop will run for 16 weeks and will consist of one weekly group session and activities for **the couples** between sessions. The facilitators will prepare topics for discussion and practice in the group sessions. Materials for the workshop can be gleaned from this book, and adapted to topics related to **couple relationships** and to the needs of the group and its members. It is recommended to introduce a lot of role-playing between the partners of each couple and between mixed couples, in order to diversify the mutual experiences and learning. The technique of changing roles during simulations will contribute to a deeper understanding of the partners in a couple relationship. Those planning the activities should consider their suitability for implementation in reality.

2. This stage allows the couples to personally experience their unique hardships in discreet conditions, with timing and at a pace suited to them. Each couple will decide for itself. The facilitator will plan the meetings to suit the needs of the couple under his care.

It is recommended to plan social meetings for the entire group once a month.

CONCLUSION AND PARTING - This stage will include a summing up discussion, mutual feedback, the facilitators' summary, a social party and plans for continued social contact between the participants.

GUIDELINES FOR THE FACILITATORS AND THERAPISTS:

The guidelines of this project are **significant**:

1. It is **advisable** that each facilitator be of a different gender, as the participants will generally be of both genders.
2. Both facilitators must have specialized and acquired experience in group therapy and in treating people with Asperger's (ASD), in addition to their experience in treating couples.
3. This is a **complex** program, from a professional standpoint: It requires therapeutic professionalism integrating three dimensions. For this reason, it is important that each facilitator can support his partner, and contribute from his accumulative knowledge and experience. The facilitators must have previous experience.
4. Take into account that preparing and establishing the group is time-consuming, therefore everything should be planned accordingly.

This project opens doors of hope, along with **realistic** optimism, for adults with Asperger's (ASD).

III – A GROUP FOR EMPOWERING PARENTS OF ADULTS WITH ASPERGER'S (ASD)

ROOTS AND WINGS

Give them roots with which to grow, and wings with which to fly and find joy.

INTRODUCTION

Parents, by their very nature, aspire to see their children grow and develop into adulthood and independence and to reach self-fulfillment. Young neurotypical adults naturally leave their parents' home upon reaching adulthood and build their personal and social lives. In contrast, parents who must cope with children with special needs, need the help of a guiding, supporting and empowering framework.

Herein lies the importance of initiating and operating groups of parents to adults with Asperger's (ASD).

ADVANTAGES OF THE GROUP:

1. Parents coping with similar uncertainties find in the group a safe and supporting milieu.
2. Encouraging connections, **openness**, cohesion, **understanding** and acceptance.
3. Support and empowerment among equals is a framework in which its members enjoy a unique opportunity for reciprocal learning. Sharing with others the different experiences facilitates mutual learning from the successes and failures of others.

4. Professional facilitation contributes to an understanding of the unique problems faced by people with Asperger's (ASD).

5. This project will provide the parents with tools and deepen their self-awareness, thus contributing to a better understanding of their son/daughter. As a result, they will be able to develop a more suitable and constructive relationship with them.

THE HUMANISTIC APPROACH IN GROUP FACILITATION
GUIDELINES FOR THE FACILITATORS

1. Create relationships between the facilitator and the participants "at eye level."

2. Listen, understand (empathy) and accept each of the group members.

3. Identify potential crisis situations and prepare accordingly.

4. Recognize your responsibility toward the group and its progress.

5. Be flexible and, when necessary, consult with colleagues.

6. Write a brief summary after each session, for later evaluation and drawing conclusions.

7. Read the program of the workshops in Part III (of this book) and implement the guidelines for facilitators.

III - A GROUP FOR EMPOWERING PARENTS OF ADULTS WITH ASPERGER'S (ASD)

A PROGRAM FOR GROUP FACILITATION OF PARENTS OF ADULTS WITH ASPERGER'S (ASD)

SESSION 1: PRELIMINARY ACQUAINTANCE

a. The facilitator introduces himself, **then** makes the rounds, asking each participant to introduce himself and his family.

b. A discussion is held on the terms of **the framework and the commitment** of the group members.

SESSION 2: DEEPENING THE ACQUAINTANCE

a. Each member brings from home an item that has meaning for him and shares with the group his dreams and ambitions, experiences and lessons learned, etc.

b. **Commitment and Confidentiality** – The facilitator presents the topic and leads **a group discussion.**

SESSION 3: THE ACHIEVEMENTS AND HARDSHIPS OF THE SON/ DAUGHTER IN THE PAST/PRESENT.

a. All the members of the group speak in turn. The facilitator demonstrates and encourages that questions be directed to the person who is speaking. He emphasizes the statement: "If we don't ask, how will we know?" – a question is the preferred tool in testing reality, rather than inconclusive assumptions.

b. A discussion on **what is similar and what is different** in our children's abilities and difficulties.

SESSION 4:

a. **Asperger's (ASD)** - **the Elusive syndrome** – the facilitator prepares a short lecture on the subject, to help the parents understand the basic nature of the syndrome, along with the causes, hardships, results and consequences of its characteristic behaviorisms.

b. **The group members** are divided into two **small groups** and discuss a topic, in light of their personal experiences, and clarify misunderstandings through asking questions. They then write down their practical conclusions regarding their everyday life. They present this before the entire group and receive the other members' reactions. The facilitator encourages a discussion.

SESSION 5:

a. **Living as an adult with the syndrome, the social ties and social difficulties** – a short lecture by the facilitator, followed by a group discussion.

b. How my child **has had to cope** over the years with harassments and pestering.

SESSION 6:

a. **Parents as mediators, supporters and reinforcers.** What do we possess that can be used to help and promote our children, what abilities and skills can be applied and recruited for them in their process of adjusting to an adult life?

b. **The parents with themselves** – what are **our** needs? A conversation led by the facilitator.

SESSION 7:

a. **Authority and boundaries in our family**. How are these perceived by the parents and by the children, and how are they expressed?

b. What can we learn from the group members on ways of affecting changes in our family. An interactive discussion, guided by the facilitator.

SESSION 8:

a. **The roles in our family** – how are they carried out? How is responsibility divided among the family members? What can be improved and how? A group discussion.

b. **Responsibility**, well-defined, determination and perseverance, routine in filling the role, maximum responsibility over the personal matters of our son/daughter. Partnership or conflict?

SESSION 9:

a. **Communication and family connections** – The facilitator prepares a short lecture on the subject, with emphasis on the communication patterns in a family that promote personal ties, openness and closeness. The group members contribute from their own experiences and relate events that happened to them. The facilitator encourages a discussion.

b. The facilitator stages simulations of events that were reported, and initiates role-playing. The members share with the group their experiences and hold a group discussion about the significance of the relationships within the family and the possibilities for improvement. The facilitator leads a discussion, clarifying the subject of the communication of the adult with Asperger's (ASD) within his family.

SESSION 10:

a. **Difficulty in expressing emotions** - reasons, processes and results. The facilitator prepares a short lecture on the subject, and briefly mentions neurological causes, a unique language of thinking and various patterns of communication. He opens the floor for questions and discussion among the members.

b. The group holds a discussion on the hardships faced by their sons/daughters with the syndrome, guided by the facilitator who indicates different ways of helping. For example: Practicing eye contact with a dialogue partner, or demonstrations and explanations of physical and verbal emotional expression. The session ends with a discussion on improving the quality of communication in order to create an efficient connection.

SESSION 11:

a. **Social isolation – Parents as advocates** for their sons/daughters with Asperger's (ASD). The discussion is devoted to issues regarding their social seclusion, the parents' involvement in raising awareness of the source of the problem, and how to use self-advocacy in social situations and in formal and informal frameworks, and building a bridge of communication with the neurotypical population in the social and employment arenas.

IDEAS FOR SELF-ADVOCACY:

1. We are not indifferent nor belittling, we simply have a hard time deciphering social cues.

2. We have a kind of "hidden blindness" that hampers our

ability to understand body language and facial expressions and their meanings.

3. We learn with the help of our intelligence, to understand what it is we don't understand and to dare **to ask** in order to move forward with communication.

4. If we rely on ourselves and learn to accept ourselves, we will be able to connect with others and give of our abilities.

All the above are topics for in-depth **discussions** in the group, from which role-playing can be created, touching upon the communication between adults with Asperger's (ASD) and neurotypical people. Via role-playing and with the facilitator's guidance, the parents can try to develop a conversation with family members or one of their children about their son/daughter with Asperger's (ASD) and the relationship within the family.

SESSION 12: CRITICISM OR FEEDBACK?

a. The ease of **confusing** between giving **feedback** and giving **criticism** or being judgmental: After a brief introduction, the facilitator engages the parents in a discussion on how they cope with their son/daughter with the syndrome. The discussion should lead to a dialogue of comparative analysis between the two situations, and their beneficial or harmful effect. **The background:** Many parents try "to correct" their children's behavior, out of concern and a **sincere** desire **to help** them. Unfortunately, the children feel hurt, as they don't understand **where they went wrong**. Therefore, this issue should be discussed in greater depth, accompanied by an analysis of incidents presented by the parents.

b. A discussion on **the principles of giving feedback**, guiding the parents as to how to use it, along with demonstrations using role-playing.

SESSION 13:

a. **To change and to affect change,** or to help our children find ways of **adjusting** to reality as it is? The facilitator presents this dilemma and invites the participants to role-play. Each couple acts out a situation in which the parent tries to influence his child to want to change. They discuss how change can take place, which is followed by a debate on the following question: "Is it possible to change without feeling confused?" Each couple presents the exercise in turn, and the observers enter their comments in their notebooks.

b. An in-depth discussion on the objective of the above experience and the **dilemma** that is concretely expressed in the role-playing. The facilitator presents possibilities that will help build a more rewarding life: Studies, preparing for employment, fitting into a workplace, a workshop for developing social life skills, social groups, preparation for couple relationships (see Parts c and d).

SESSION 14:

a. **Two different languages of thought** – a situation that gives rise to misunderstandings that disrupt communication and repeatedly lead to further misunderstandings. The facilitator briefly explains this phenomenon, which obstructs people with Asperger's (ASD) to connect with others and adjust. The parents' contribution can be along several lines:

1. Exercises in identifying and deciphering their son/daughter's experiences.

2. Practicing what the other person's intentions and feelings are.

3. Focusing on what are the codes and behavioral norms in social situations.

4. Encouraging the son/daughter to join social groups and workshops for developing social life skills.

b. **Practicing a conversation** between a parent and his adult offspring with Asperger's (ASD), discussing the cooperation between them. At first, the son/daughter rejects the suggestion, and the parent continues, trying to cope with the refusal. Following this, the facilitator leads a discussion in the **group forum**, after each "parent" experiences a conversation with the "refusing son/daughter."

1. At this stage, the parent and child role-players provide feedback to one another.

2. The observers discuss what took place during this experience, and provide feedback to the role-players.

SESSION 15:

a. **Summing up:** The goal of this session is to create a transition stage between what the parents have learned and actually applying or implementing it with their child. The group members receive guidance from the facilitator as to how to plan support, encouragement and cooperation, and **write down** his suggestions in their journals. Following that, each parent (or parental couple) writes out a plan of action that is suitable to his family.

b. Each one reads out his plan and explains the rationale behind the choices he made and the details about his family that he took into account. This is done by all the members, by turn, and the others respond with questions and comments. The facilitator intervenes when needed.

SESSION 16: SUMMING UP AND PARTING

a. A **concluding** discussion on the learning process that the parents prepared in writing – what have they received, what have they learned, what can they apply to their own lives, and how does all this affect the family and the adults with Asperger's (ASD?

b. Parting – Each member of the group prepares a written or oral feedback for each of the other members or couples. The **rationale** of this process is: Everyone has gotten to know the others, and the parting gift will be to give them information or a reflection that will help them and **empower** them in the future.

c. The facilitator suggests that the group members continue meeting together once in a while, and keep in touch with one another. He invites the participants to respond, and recommends a permanent forum to help the parents share and receive support, and proposes a farewell party at the home of one of the couples.

IV – SELF-HELP

CHAPTER 1: Self-Help for the Adult with Asperger's (ASD) – Survival and Growth in the Neurotypical World

"Within each of us great forces are hidden, we need only discover them and use them."
David Ben-Gurion

INTRODUCTION

"Most of our mistakes are caused by the fact that we still don't understand the 'Aspergerian' (ASD) language." These words were spoken by one of the therapists, working to find ways to rehabilitate people with Asperger's (ASD). This key sentence reflects the complexity of their lives, in a world conducted via neurotypical thought and communication language, which adults with the syndrome find hard to decipher. As a result, they remain strangers within their culture and community and seclude themselves. Two adults with Asperger's (ASD), Edmonds and Worton (2006), wrote a personal guidebook in which they give tips on how to cope in the various areas of life in a world not designed for them. In order to demonstrate the influence of the environment on successful (or unsuccessful) coping, they relate the virtual life story of identical twins with the syndrome. Even though both were equally talented and their minds worked in identical ways, their development was totally different. The twin who was raised by supportive parents was able to overcome his difficulties and succeeded, whereas his brother who was raised separately by judgmental parents, developed a low self-image and was unsuccessful.

The differences in thinking patterns and communication among adults diagnosed with Asperger's (ASD) and neurotypical adults (a sample):

a. The point of departure when looking to the welfare of adults with Asperger's (ASD) is the approach that relates to **each individual as a whole person**, and focuses on ways of coping that are **unique to him**.

b. Adults with Asperger's (ASD) **must neither give up, nor give in to stereotypes,** yet at the same time they **mustn't get angry at the ignorance of others**, as even for those of good will, the communication with them may be confusing.

c. Lovett (2005) emphasizes **the difference** between people with the syndrome and neurotypical people, in the manner in which **information is processed**. Adults with Asperger's (ASD) tend to discern the important details along with the less important details, as they excel in **remembering details**. Neurotypical people are structured to gather details selectively, which together will lead them to **deciphering the meaning** of an event by perceiving the wider picture. Frith (1991) named this "central coherence" which, as said, typifies neurotypical people and is lacking in those with Asperger's (ASD). Becoming **aware** of this impediment opens the way to begin better communication.

d. Lovett (2005) claims that the difficulty for people with the syndrome in the **manageable functionality** of their everyday life is also related to a weak central coherence. Functioning is based on **cognitive flexibility**, which is required in order to examine options and to identify what is important, unimportant or impractical in any given situation. The **pragmatic** way of thinking enables one to learn from experience and adjust his **behavior, based on feedback from the given situation**. Efficient functioning includes, inter alia, a correct use of the accepted rules in a **specific situation**, consolidating a clear goal, and constancy in taking steps toward that goal. Adults with the syndrome find it hard to organize their actions and carry them out efficiently, especially when faced with new challenges, and it stands to reason that these difficulties are also influenced by the problem of **central coherence**. Lovett (2005) sums up the subject with a question that expresses what neurotypical people think about the difficulty in understanding those diagnosed with Asperger's (ASD): How is it possible that someone that looks so intelligent and capable has so many problems in dealing with life?". **This contradiction** is frequently interpreted as selfishness or negativity, and therefore **arouses anger** among the neurotypical partners.

e.   An additional link in the chain of hardships, which adds further complexity to a relationship, is the difficulty of those diagnosed with Asperger's (ASD) to understand what is taking place in the other person's mind. Many of them lack the ability to "read the mind" of the other, a phenomenon which Baron-Cohen (1995) named "mental blindness." Lovett (2005) proposes two basic general rules that, if implemented, will facilitate the communication between those with the syndrome and neurotypical people. She holds that at the base of the communication, the adult with Asperger's (ASD) must possess a **self-awareness** of his difficulties and, along with that, the **neurotypical partner must have awareness** of his partner's problems within this connection. The basis for communication between them will be this meeting of two different thinking patterns. These basic postulations will prevent surprises, frustrations and anger on both sides. Thus, the neurotypical person will know to phrase what he means precisely, and why he must do so, and the adult with the syndrome will be aware that he must ask his dialogue partner what he means exactly and why it is important. This awareness will minimize the "mental blindness" that arises from the different patterns of thinking.

f.   It is generally held among therapists that supporting people with Asperger's (ASD) **must focus** on the manner in which they interpret the world, with emphasis on logic, and practical, structured thinking. Nonetheless, one must keep in mind that their deficiency, manifested in their difficulty in identifying, naming and expressing emotions, is a critical factor in their personal and social life. Thus, adults with the syndrome should be taught to understand, identify and categorize the diversity of emotions in a way that can shift from the cognitive to the experiential and emotional, and then back to logical thought. From my clinical experience in both individual and group therapy, this method brought significant benefit. By doing so, we are utilizing the cognitive skills in order to help adults with the syndrome overcome the deficiency in understanding their feelings and in their ability to communicate.

g.   Lovett (2005) presents a number of options for self-help:

1.   Maintaining a personal diary of events, in which the writer describes everything that **took place** at an event

and **what he experienced**.

2. An in-depth observation of what is happening at an event, and an attempt to define the **connection** between what **is happening** to what he **is feeling**.

3. Trying to reconstruct previous events that were experienced, and draw conclusions from them on the connection between one's behavior and its consequences.

4. Check oneself to see if he conducted himself in an accepted manner and if there is a better way.

5. Reading the diary of events on a regular basis, when fully relaxed.

6. Learning to smile – smiling is the most important emotional gesture in interaction. Practice smiling in front of a mirror.

7. Receiving feedback on personal exercises from people he depends on.

8. Practicing various emotions in front of a mirror, exercising facial expressions in order to learn how to express emotions beyond the spoken word.

9. Learning how to cope with an overload of emotions by breathing deeply, relaxing and doing whatever calms him down.

h. Edmonds et al (2006) address the issues of over-sensitivity, distress and emotional overload. They suggest some tips for coping with these situations:

1. Discuss the problem with someone **you believe in.**

2. Explain to others your special needs and help them accept this!

3. Immerse yourself in something totally different, such as a hobby, etc.

4. Channel the energies of anger into a different direction, such as physical activity!

5. **Channel** the energy to something that **will help** someone else in a positive way!

6. Don't be harsh with yourself and **be proud** that you tried to do your best!

7. **Self-empowerment** - by **rising above** the angering factor, and above the words and actions of the other person and yourself.

8. **Praise yourself for coping** with social isolation, and appreciate yourself for not giving up.

9. **Do not give in** to frustration because of interpersonal failure, continue constantly and persistently. What doesn't kill you - **toughens you.**

i. Lovett (2005) also addresses such phenomena as anxiety and depression. Difficulties in coping with the neurotypical world give rise to anxieties and a sense of failure, hopelessness and helplessness, which lead to depression. Experiences of rejection also lead to frustration and depression. These are all negative emotions **that take their toll** on the health of people with the syndrome. She suggests some ways of coping:

1. Be **physically active** as a way of life.

2. Listen to **relaxing music** that you love.

3. Maintain your **health** and optimal **body weight**.

4. Get involved in a relaxing activity, such as walking along the beach, etc.

5. Try to explain to neurotypical people that you have difficulty in deciphering the feelings of others as well as yourself. Explain that **anger is more confusing**, but if they **explain themselves** calmly, clearly and quietly, the adult

with the syndrome will also **gain by being understood**.

j.   People with Asperger's (ASD) find it hard **to take risks**. The roots of this problem are to be found in **a fear of change**, failure and loss of control. In contrast, when opposition to change weakens and a person with the syndrome **is open** to accepting encouragement, he can learn how to **contain** a situation of both **risk and chance**, and make his **life** more colorful and **satisfying. How can you begin to feel comfortable with the idea of trying something new?** Lovett suggests:

1.   Ask yourself, what is **the worst-case scenario**?

2.   If the worst happens, what can be done and who can you turn to for **help?**

3.   Remind yourself that getting used to something new is **naturally difficult** for everyone.

k.   It is important to point out those steps that will promote the personal well-being of the adult with the syndrome. The basis is that the adult with the syndrome and the people around him understand that Asperger's (ASD) is a syndrome that plays **a major role** in his life, but it does not **define** his entire **personality**. The person with the syndrome and his supporters will do well to focus on **ways** for him **to cope successfully**. People with the syndrome sometimes feel hurt by the lack of understanding from professionals and members of their community. This author **suggests** not to accept the widespread ignorance in this matter, but also not to get angry. Instead, **help** should be offered to create a friendly culture **through clarifications and explanations**. The following are examples of contentions that grow out of a lack of understanding: "If only you'd try harder," or "You're not flexible, you're even intentionally stubborn." The **effort** made by the adult with Asperger's (ASD) to adjust is **exhausting** and may lead to **outbursts** or even a breakdown. Therefore, it is **important** that he possess the tools with which **to calm himself!**

l. The author suggests to whoever was diagnosed with Asperger's (ASD) to **arrange for himself** a place with a **friendly ambiance** and where his needs are understood, a place where **he can be himself**. Additional factors that should be attended to are relaxation, sleeping well, healthy **eating habits**, **physical** activity, taking medications regularly, and a good **understanding** of the accompanying emotional problems and the best way **to handle** them.

m. Pay attention to the bipolar way of thinking - in terms of **black or white** - of adults with the syndrome, and to their desire to examine situations **logically.** Take into account that there aren't always clear-cut answers in this manner of thinking, especially in social and interpersonal fields. **Flexible thinking** is an art that can be acquired through practice. However, many adults with the syndrome are constantly preoccupied with intellectual thinking, driven by a need **to decipher** the world. Following are some steps that can be taken to break the "thinking trap":

1. Make an effort to think **positive** thoughts.
2. Try to create images that will help you feel good.
3. Consistently convince yourself that you control **your mind,** and believe that positive thoughts will generate good feelings.
4. Appreciate yourself for changes you succeeded in doing and document your accomplishments.

5. **Don't compare** yourself to others – it is frustrating and leads to jealousy, anger and bitterness.
6. Check the possibilities for getting help through empowering therapies and **pet-assisted therapy.**

In conclusion, we wish to reiterate that the **different way of thinking** of people with Asperger's (ASD) can be **very creative** and can enrich us all when we let it flower in an accepting and encouraging environment.

IV – SELF-HELP

CHAPTER 2: SELF-HELP FOR THE ADULT WITH ASPERGER'S (ASD) – APPROACHING OTHERS IN SOCIAL SITUATIONS

Be one who loves people, and respect them honestly and prudently

INTRODUCTION FOR THE FACILITATOR

People with Asperger's (ASD) experience the social world as an elusive maze in which it is hard to find one's way. Many of them yearn for social contact, even though they harbor a certain withdrawal from interpersonal communication, following past frustrating attempts.

This chapter was written under the inspiration of the book by Edmonds et al (2006), *The Asperger Social Guide*. In their introduction to the book, they remind us that every person during the course of his day-to-day life is confronted with a wide variety of social situations, some of which are experienced as a mine field of embarrassment and confusion. The rules of social conduct are usually learned naturally by neurotypical people, whereas for a person with the syndrome, this is a difficult task, as social behavior includes pragmatic thinking that is based on its context, such as: culture, norms, framework, timing, the nature of the interpersonal connection, etc.

The authors suggest tips for the reader to consider and apply, to help him cope in a more effective way.

ONE SMILE LEADS TO ANOTHER – POSITIVE THINKING

a. Whoever has had to absorb negative treatment from others because he doesn't behave as most other do, must not let his spirit drop, as most people **are fixated** on the accepted ways of behavior and find it hard to understand behavior that is different.

b. Adults with Asperger's (ASD) approach life logically, and this is a relative advantage.

c. The greater your self-acceptance, the easier it will be for others to accept you.

d. Refraining from comparisons with others and **focusing on your own abilities and achievements** will prepare you for positive adjustment.

e. The effort to be **positive** will help you in the process of integrating into the neurotypical society.

f. Remember that those who tease you are the ones with the low self-image. **Do not** be tempted to internalize the humiliations and create a negative image of yourself.

g. Focus on your talents and **your strengths!!!**

h. **Empathy** is the basis for gaining successful treatment from others, and you must trust your **instincts**. It is therefore recommended that you make every effort to develop in that direction.

i. The social milieu doesn't react politely to public outbursts, especially outbursts of frustration and anger. The correct way to handle these emotions is via **consultation** or with the help of anyone who serves as a **supporting figure** for you.

WAYS OF APPROACHING OTHERS – PRACTICAL TIPS

a. **Relating** is the ability to socially communicate with other people. It is expressed in the exchange of information **in a manner suited to the person and the situation**. This means that thought and learning should be invested in relating to others, finding the way **that suits you best** and applying it.

b. **Communication by phone** – Prepare what you want to say in writing to decrease your anxiety. Most people are pleasant. Whoever is impatient, it is **his problem**; one can assume that he treats **others** as well in the same way.

c. **Conversation** is based on both verbal and non-verbal communication. In order to develop conversational skills, you should **practice,** and learn how to communicate in a manner that you find **comfortable.**

d. **Tips for conversation** –Learn to speak **in turn: Don't monopolize** the conversation, allow others to join in, **ask them** what they would like to add. Learn how to **observe non-verbal cues:** Is your dialogue partner looking sideways or frequently checking the time? This may be due to boredom or a lack of time. Pay attention also to the circumstances in which the conversation is taking place – they are not always obvious.

e. **Eye contact** – As much as possible, it is important to look at your dialogue partner from time to time.

f. **Joining in** – it is important to know **when is the right time** or not the time to **join in** the conversation of others. If you know the other people, you usually can join in. It is always **better to ask**: Is this a private conversation or can I join in?

g. **Tone of voice** – It is recommended that you become **aware** of the importance of this. Try to **adjust** your tone of voice to the **context** of the conversation: A high-pitched voice to express joy, a quiet voice to express sadness. **Do not be crass** – it may hurt others and lead to their pulling away. Try to introduce **humor** into your conversation.

h. **Questions** – Adults with Asperger's (ASD) **tend to ask a lot of questions** on a daily basis, as a means of **deciphering the** confusing neurotypical **world.** At times, this is a good method for coping that promotes individual development. On the other hand, it is recommended **to develop control and proportionality** by frequently checking **the listener's reaction.**

i. **Showing interest** – People with the syndrome tend to talk about a topic that interests them, however the neurotypical listener doesn't like to hear the same thing over and over again; try to **touch upon a variety of subjects**. Remember, what you find exciting may not necessarily excite others.

j. **Ending the conversation** – If you are **limited in time, say so a few minutes before:** "I'm sorry to interrupt you, however I must leave," or "I hope we can continue this next time we meet."

k. **Listening – eye contact** is a **basic** rule. If you find this hard, glance at the other person from time to time. Be aware of your body language, pay attention that you don't appear bored, that you don't yawn or look at your watch etc. it can be misconstrued as an insult. To prevent this, explain to your dialogue partner the reason for this. **You are expected** to be polite and **to listen,** just as **you expect this** from others.

l. **Non-verbal listening** – Due to the difficulties experienced by those diagnosed with Asperger's (ASD) to decipher social situations, as well as intentions and thoughts, it is recommended to ask for clarification: "I'd be grateful if you could speak to me as directly and clearly as possible." You should do this in situations in which it is truly important to you to understand **the significance** of what is being said.

m. **Instructions** – it is especially **important to listen** to instructions. You can ask for further **clarifications** or suggest that the other person speak more slowly to allow you to write down what he is saying. Since you are obligated to agree with the one giving instructions and **to carry them out, you are responsible for getting clarifications** and fulfilling the instructions successfully.

n. **Help or advice** – Adults with Asperger's (ASD) are good listeners. At times others will share their feelings with them, out of their need to talk to someone, yet they do not expect advice or answers in return. It is sufficient **to show them** that you **understand** them and **you are sincerely listening to them.**

o. **Auditory understanding** – Listening to people with a foreign accent is hard at times. During meaningful conversations it is important to listen attentively – this promotes building a connection and maintaining it. **It is customary** to ask the dialogue partner to repeat what he has said in order to **understand completely**. Highly recommended!

p. **Processing data** – it is most important to find an efficient way to process media-reported data. It opens the door to good **communication in the long run.**

q. **Humor** – Spontaneous **humor** to create **social ties.** People with the syndrome have a sense of humor too, except that it is different. Thus, think well if you are about to **express** your brand of humor before **the right people**. Additionally, learn **not to feel personally hurt by cynical humor**. Try to **connect positively,** and say: "I'm sure you didn't mean to hurt anyone by that."

r. **Harassment** – People who are socially **naïve** are targets for harassment. Do not minimize your ability to be **assertive!** Nothing justifies harassment, and no one deserves such treatment ever. **It is recommended** that you recognize your **strengths** and utilize them, in order to **demand** assertively the **respect** you deserve. And don't let harassments **frighten** you. it is good to **ask for help,** as needed.

s. **Tips for being properly treated in every situation** – no one, a neurotypical person or someone different, is able to express himself or read the other person's non-verbal language **perfectly**. "All non-verbal social communication is a matter of impressions and interpretation and is open for discussion, as it cannot be measured" (Edmonds and Worton, 2006).

t. **Smiling** – A smile is a gesture that in the long run brings compensation. A smile transmits the desire for good, pleasant relationships with hope for reciprocity. This gesture is of great importance!

u. **Calling by name** – Mentioning the name of your dialogue partner creates the feeling that you are relating to him personally, and this has a **good impact** on the communication between you!

v. **Be accessible** – Adults with Asperger's (ASD) do not demonstrate their feelings externally, therefore it is desirable to practice this, and **receive feedback** from people that you **rely on**. Social anxiety leads to emotional withdrawal. Try **"opening"** your body's posture and **face your dialogue partner**. This increases the feeling of your accessibility to others.

w. **Physical space** – Standing **too close** can be misconstrued as **invasiveness** or aggressiveness. In contrast, standing **too far away transmits a lack of interest** or hesitation in social situations.

x. **Demonstrate involvement** by confirming with a nod of your head, through eye contact and phrases such as: "I understand," "I really didn't know that," "Really?," "Wow!," "Oh, no!," "Thank God," etc., that are **appropriate** to the context of the conversation.

y. **Greetings** – keep in mind the significance of greetings such as "Hello," "See you soon," "It was nice meeting you," etc. This is an expression of politeness, kindness and **friendliness toward others**.

z. **Be aware of the feelings of others** – Learn **to ask** while talking with another: "What's your opinion on that?," "How do you feel about it?," etc. It will **help you learn** how others feel. Don't exaggerate and **don't ask a lot of questions**.

aa. **Think outside yourself** – It is easy to be drawn into focusing on yourself and forgetting to focus on others. **The ability to relate to others** calms anxieties, **increases self-confidence** and lowers the level of tension.

ab. **Small talk** – Try to **learn** methods for creating small talk. The basic principle is to learn to relate not only to information, but also to the **relationships** in the interactive process, such as: "Don't worry, what's going on now will remain only between us," "I understand you, I've experienced something similar," "Let's talk about what we've learned from this experience," etc.

ac. **Trust in others** – it is worthwhile the effort **to try to trust** others. **This is the only way** to relate positively to those with whom we want to be in touch with.

ad. **A willingness to help** –a sincere desire to help is always **received positively.** This is proof that you are of goodwill and want **to develop positive relationships**. Be careful that you

don't agree to every suggestion, just to be liked. The ability to say that you are unable to accommodate the request is acceptable. It is important **to refuse politely**, such as: "I'm sorry, but this time it won't work out" (with a smile), etc.

ae. **Accept your social limitations, and search for support.** You are **worthy of it.** You have the right to fight to get support, and you are responsible for finding a way **to implement it**!!!

EPILOGUE

Adults with Asperger's (ASD) experience reality differently from neurotypical people. The difference derives from their unique neurological functioning and is manifested mainly in their difficulty to understand, to adjust, to fit in and to navigate their life as adults, and this impacts their limited ability to decipher social and interpersonal codes. They need professional help that will impart the necessary tools with which to cope with these and other challenges.

Adults with the syndrome experienced throughout their growing-up years repeated criticism of their strange behavior, and harsh experiences of painful rejection have been branded into their memory, which forced them to protect themselves by withdrawing. Though adults with high-level functioning have good verbal ability, they lack the skills required for maintaining effective communication and developing meaningful ties with others. This situation undermines their ability to create a reciprocal relationship and maintain long-term relationships.

Apparently, the developmental profile of an adult with the syndrome is different from that of a neurotypical adult. However, current clinical experience indicates that professional help and the support of parents, friends and significant others in the life of an adult with the syndrome can help improve his social adjustment in different frameworks.

A tolerant approach in an accepting environment will enable a person with the syndrome to feel free to be himself, and it is in precisely these conditions that he will find it easier to open himself up toward change.

This book is based on group facilitation workshops with a special emphasis on developing social life skills. This method facilitates empowerment and personal development together with a peer group, which provides social learning conditions throughout. In addition, attention is given to individual therapy as per the needs of each individual.

This book is an accompanying guide to group facilitators and therapists, and provides tools that were designed for the population of adults with the syndrome. At the same time, it also addresses parents, educators and whoever is interested in Asperger's (ASD), and constitutes an additional echelon in the efforts to advance this unique population.

APPENDIX OF PHOTOGRAPHS

ACTORS:
YISRAEL GURION
NATALIE NE'EMAN

PHOTOGRAPHER: GIDEON BAIDA

With deep gratitude for the cooperation, high-quality
implementation, and superb results

PART III – FIRST WORKSHOP
SKILLS IN EMOTIONAL COMMUNICATION (SESSIONS: 3,4,5,6)

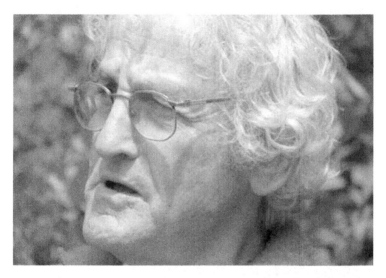

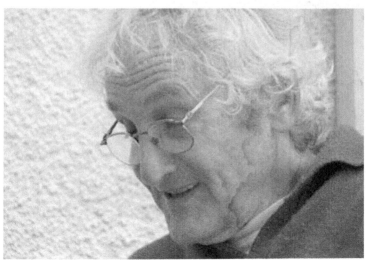

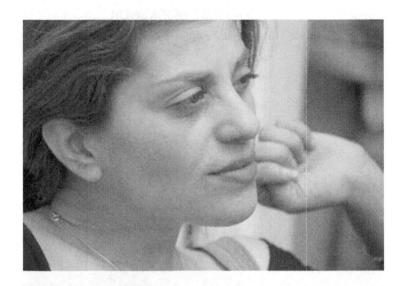

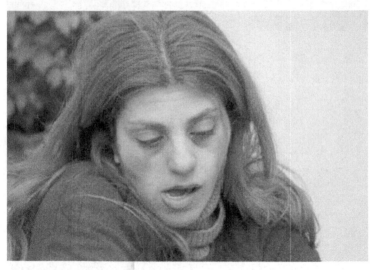

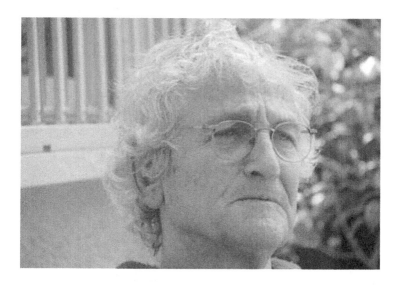

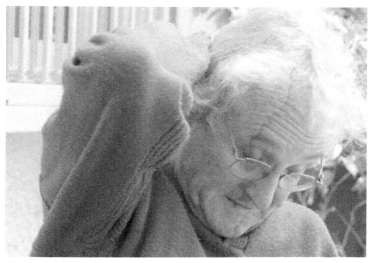

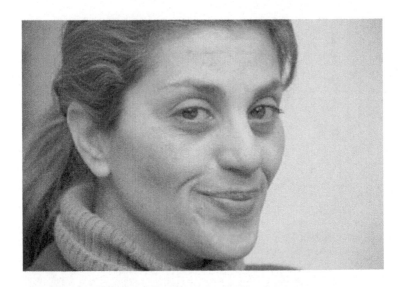

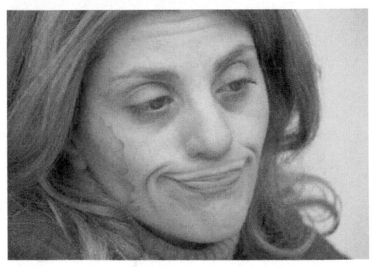

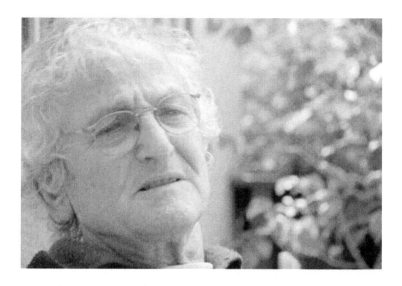

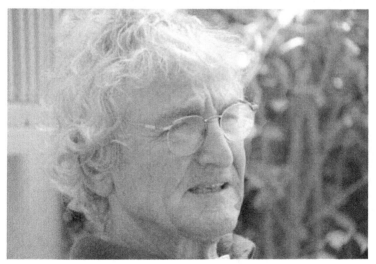

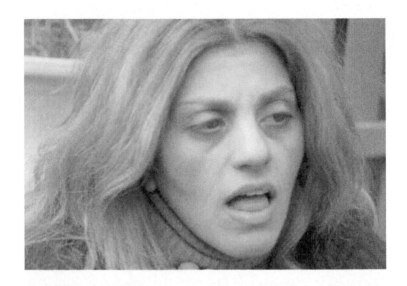

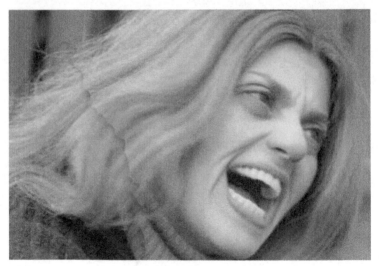

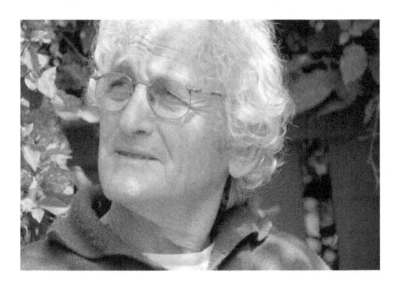

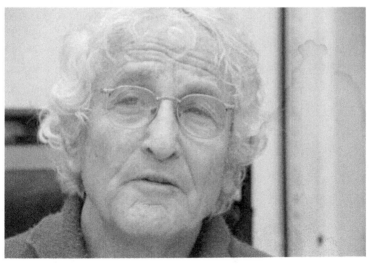

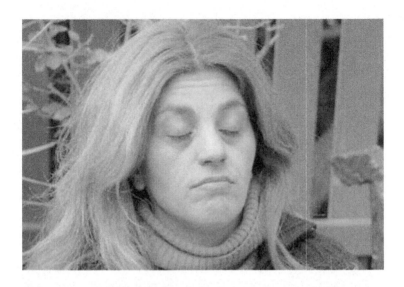

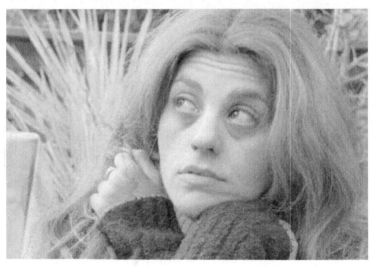

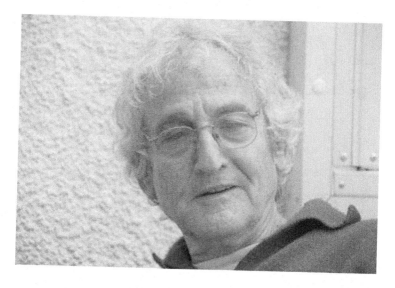

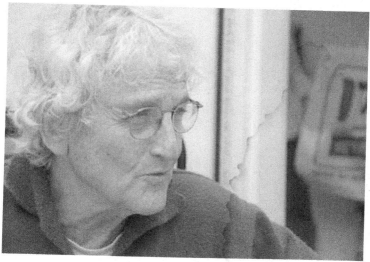

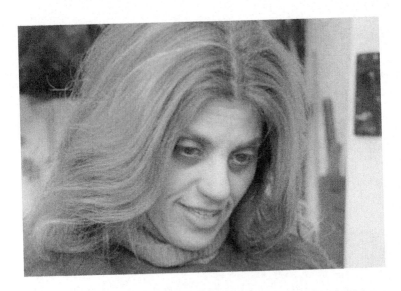

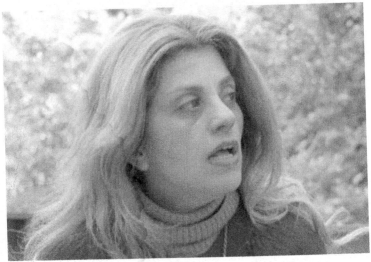

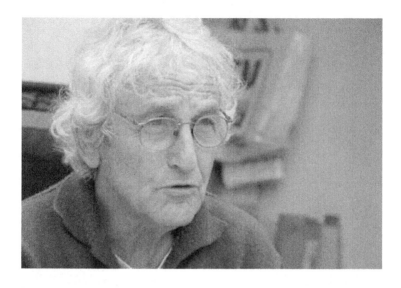

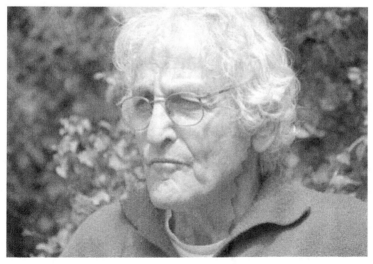

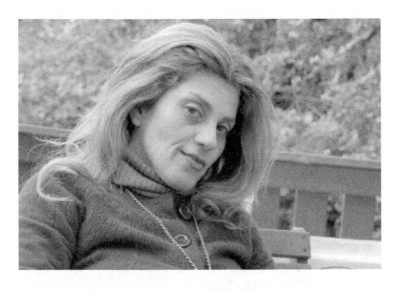

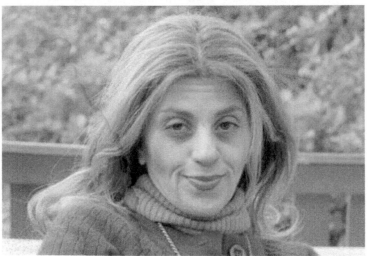

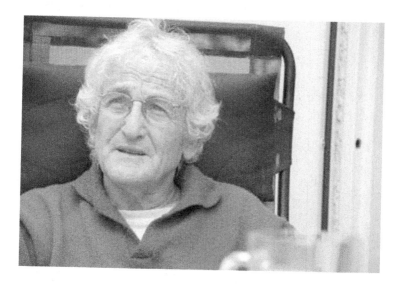

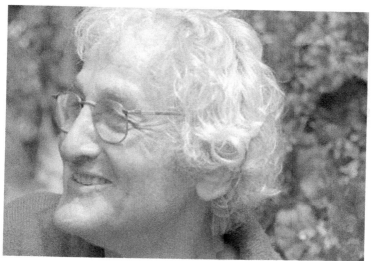

PART IV — BEING IN A COUPLE RELATIONSHIP
WITH ASPERGER'S (ASD)

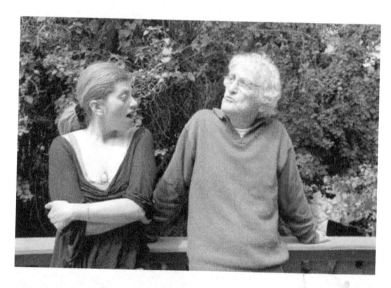

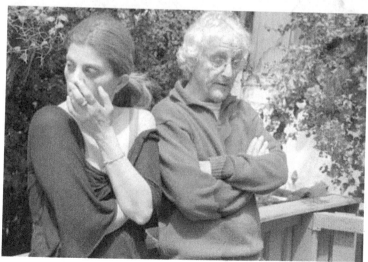

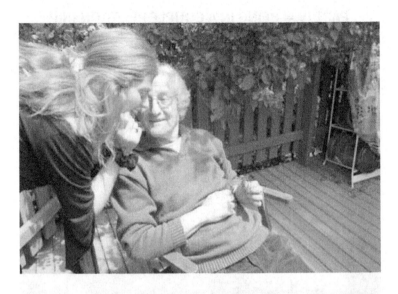

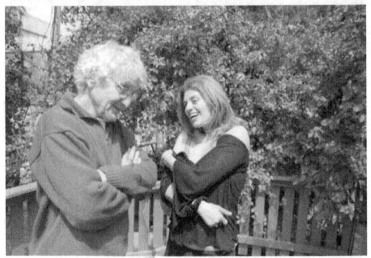

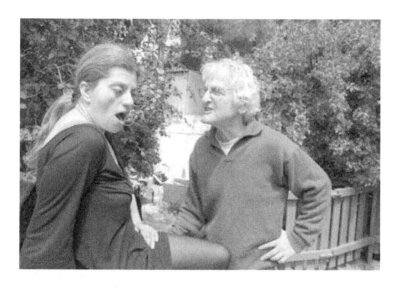

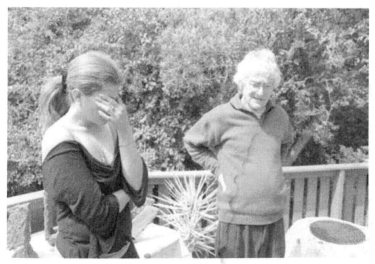

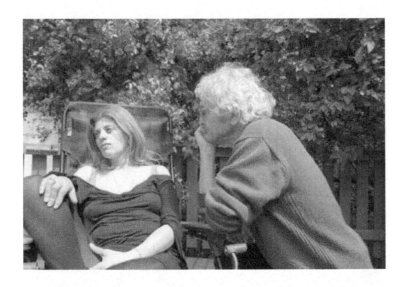

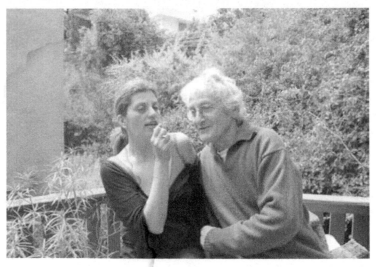

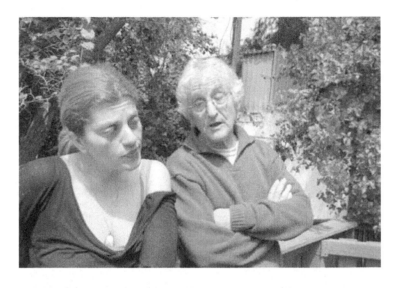

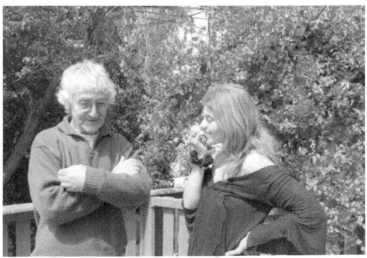

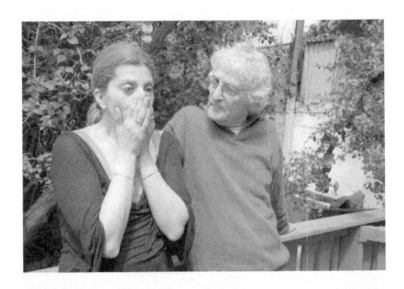

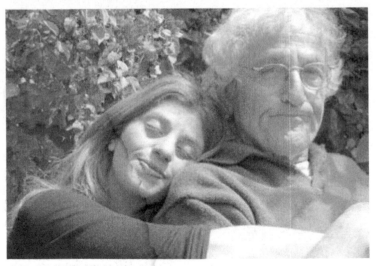

ADDENDUM FOR FACILITATORS AND THERAPISTS

INTRODUCTION

This addendum is a compendium of descriptions of the difficulties and behavior patterns characteristic of people with Asperger's (ASD), written for those involved in the rehabilitation of adults with the syndrome. It may be used prior to, following or during consultations and therapy sessions (individual or group).

Reviewing these lists will help to understand the unfamiliar behavioral traits and provide reminders and tips to assist therapists prepare for whatever treatment sessions they choose.

The lists do not include all the adversities and obstacles, as there are countless phenomena that may be similar or different. Nonetheless, each adult's personal profile is unique, comprising the difficulties and strengths that are distinctive to him. Thus, the tips in these lists comprise only a sampling.

THANKS TO THE DIAGNOSIS

A professional diagnosis is of major significance toward the acceptance, as well as conscious and emotional consolidation, of one's personal identity, and serves as a basis for the individual's readiness to enter a rehabilitation process. Adults with the syndrome all typically share the difficulty in connecting with and integrating into society, despite their excellent cognitive abilities.

Concurrently, each individual adult **is different** from the others in his personality, life experience, viewpoints and internalized values.

412 | Benjamina Eran

An adult with the syndrome finds it difficult to decipher the social situation he is confronted with and finds it hard to fit in. This impacts on other life aspects (social, occupational and family), especially in today's dynamic, intensive and changing reality. These circumstances are demanding for each one of us, but so much the more so for those adults who find it hard to cope with changes and uncertainty.

Emphasis should be put on offering understanding, acceptance and support to the parents, and diagnosis is the tool with which they can learn to understand the special needs of their son/daughter and help them make their way in a manner that bears results.

THE CHAIN OF DIFFICULTIES

1. **Relative lateness** in personal and **social** maturation.
2. A low **self-image** in the wake of a sense of failure in human relations.
3. **A perception of self** that is not consolidated and is at times negative due to a plethora of criticisms and judgmental reactions from the community.
4. **The negative reactions** are born of parental or educational devotion and concern, yet the person with the syndrome is unable to understand in what he was mistaken, leading to greater confusion and anxiety.
5. **Difficulty in understanding his own feelings** and those of others and the inability to conceptualize and communicate them.
6. **Difficulty in envisioning the results** of his behavior or that of others.
7. **Inability to replicate** the results of interaction from a current situation to a future situation.

8. **A limited understanding** of codes of reciprocal behavior in a relationship, in both the emotional and practical dimensions.
9. **Difficulty in deciphering** what Is unfolding in the mind of his dialogue partner (thoughts, **feelings**, intentions, etc., the result being – a limited capacity for empathy).
10. **Loneliness and its consequences** – repeated experiences of loneliness and exclusion.
11. **A high level of vulnerability** in the mental, functional and health dimensions.
12. **Withdrawal** and avoidance – a means of defending oneself out of fear of social failure.
13. **A desire to decipher** what is taking place, expressed by multiple repetitions of the same questions, and a tendency to talk at length about his favorite subject.
14. **Difficulty in showing interest** in others, in initiating, being spontaneous, etc.
15. **A fear of change**, even the slightest one, in circumstances, people, location, etc.
16. **Disconnecting** or daydreaming while in conversation or in the presence of others.
17. A high or low sensitivity to sensory stimuli (heat, cold, noise, odors, touch, etc.).
18. A rigid choice of foods and clothing.
19. Exaggerated reactions to distractions while concentrating.
20. Self management (time, responsibility, organizing items, activities, etc.).

COGNITIVE BEHAVIORAL CHARACTERISTICS

1. **Standard intelligence** (average), high or even greater.
2. **A tendency to interpret** verbal messages or statements literally.

3. **Difficulty in understanding** instructions and training **and difficulty in understanding** humor and perceiving cues (body and facial expressions).
4. **Preference** for detailed instructions (step by step).
5. **Repeating the same question** several times as a mechanism to reduce anxiety, due to an inability to decipher the "social map."
6. **Making decisions** and solving problems that is different from the accepted way.
7. **Intensive interest** in a specific area and trifling involvement in other areas.
8. **Giving attention to small details**, beyond the usual.
9. **Difficulty in understanding** the rules of reciprocity and cooperation.
10. **A lack of initiative** and spontaneity.
11. **Impulsiveness** and difficulty in regulating emotions.
12. **Difficulty with short-term memory**, attention and concentration.

SOCIAL CHARACTERISTICS

1. **Difficulty in internalizing** and applying unwritten norms and social rules that are accepted and practiced in society-at-large.
2. **Difficulty in self-management** vis-à-vis authority (failure in reading the social map).
3. **Suspiciousness** on the one hand and naivety on the other hand – toward strangers.
4. **Rigidity in interaction** or negotiation to reinforce a sense of control.
5. **Difficulty in differentiating** between a companion, friend or acquaintance.

6. **Lack of clarity** as to boundaries in relationships (personal space).

7. **Accretion** of hurtful experiences and their long-term effect.

8. **Seclusion, high vulnerability** and sensitivity. Anger, sometimes outbursts, that remain unclarified to the others present.

9. **Anxiety and depression** that grow out of loneliness and a low self-image.

10. **Disturbance - in attention span and concentration** – as an impediment in organization, in "flowing" communication; a tendency toward passivity or impulsiveness (such as interrupting someone while he is speaking).

PROVIDING SKILLS AND TOOLS FOR SOCIAL ADAPTATION

1. The client's acceptance and containment as a point of departure toward developing a process of change.

2. Escorting and supporting the client by a beneficial persona.

3. Providing the client with support and guidance that help mediate between him and his neurotypical environment.

4. Follow-up and help in the aftermath of social mistakes, and counseling on how they can be resolved in interpersonal communication.

5. Providing tools for acceptable behaviorisms in various circumstances that are customary in human relations.

6. Help in acquiring an awareness of cultivating responses (initiative, giving, understanding, reciprocity, etc.).

7. Tools to cope with prejudice, harassment, insults and slander in all forms.

FROM SURVIVAL TO DEVELOPMENT – SELF-EMPOWERMENT

1. **Motivation** – high motivation to learn how to decipher the neurotypical world.

2. **Implementing exercises** in reality-testing and context evaluation in an interpersonal setting or event.

3. **To aspire toward and invest in** expanding self-awareness.

4. **Accepting the syndrome** as part of who you are and internalizing its meaning for life.

5. **Defining and appreciating** the abilities, talents and skills and other positive assets of one's personality.

6. **To practice and adopt** the habit of smiling and humor as a key to positive connections.

7. **Release restraints** and be spontaneous.

8. **Be assertive** –display a significant presence and standing on your rights, in a pleasant and non-aggressive manner.

9. **Develop a dialogue** with yourself, connecting mind and feelings.

10. **Recruit a passion** and determination for self progress and improving your coping abilities.

11. **Seek out counseling,** advice, support and help from an authorized figure, and act according to your needs and abilities, giving genuine attention to what you have been taught.

12. **Show understanding** of the fact that the purpose of all the above is to help you affect a change and improve, **but with no intention of causing you to change.**

PARENTS

Parents' denial and rejection of the diagnosis: "My son/daughter is brilliant, likes to talk, excels in school," etc.

The sons/daughters are in need of a comprehensive and professional intervention, in light of their social failures, based on understanding the necessity for a unique response to their special needs, and which does not come from anger or punishment, which only serves to further minimize his sense of self-worth.

The social deficiencies are fully laid bare when the young person with the syndrome is exposed to the demands of adolescence.

From the perspective of adult life, it is possible to discern whether a support system- or lack of it - in childhood and during adolescence influenced their preparing for adulthood.

REFERENCES

Albrecht, K. **(2010)** Social Intelligence, The New Science of

Atwood, T. **(2007)** The Complete Guide to Asperger's Syndrome. London: Jessica Kingsley Publishers

Atwood, T. **(2008)** Is There a Difference between Asperger's Syndrome and High-Functioning Autism? Retrieved Feb. 10, 2018, from http://www.tonyattwood.com.au/books-by-tony-m/resource-papers/69-is-there-a-difference-between-aspergerssyndrome-and-high-functioning-autism.

Baker, J. **(2005)** Preparing for Life, Arlington Texas: Future .Horizon Inc.

Barker, E. T., Hartley, S. L., Seltzer, M. M., Floyd, F. J., Greenberg, J. S. & Orsmond, G. I. **(2011)** Trajectories of Emotional Well-Being in Mothers of Adolescents and Adults with Autism. Developmental Psychology, 47: 551-561

Barnhill, G. **(2016)** Supporting Students with Asperger Syndrome on College Campuses: Current Practices. Focus on Autism and Other Developmental Disabilities, 31(1): 3-15. DOI: 10.1177/1088357614523121

Baron-Cohen, S., Cosmides, R. & Tooby, J. **(1995)** Mind Blindness: An Essay on Autism and Theory of Mind, Mass.: MIT Press

Baron-Cohen, S. & Wheelwright, S. **(2004)** The Empathy Quotient: An Investigation of Adults with Asperger Syndrome or High-Functioning Autism, and Normal Sex Differences. Journal of .Autism and Developmental Disorders, **34(2): 163-175**

Baron-Cohen, S. & Lai, M. C. **(2015)** Identifying The Lost Generation of Adults with Autism Spectrum Conditions. Lancet. Psychiatry, **2 (11) 1013-1027**

Benson, P. R. & Karlof, K. L. **(2009)** Anger, Stress Proliferation, and Depressed Mood among Parents of Children with ASD: A Longitudinal Replication. Journal of Autism and Developmental Disorders, **39: 350-362**

Beyer. J. F. **(2009)** Autism Spectrum Disorders and Sibling Relationships: Research and Strategies. Education and Training in Developmental Disabilities, **44: 444-452**

Bruggink A., Huisman, S., Vuijkc, R., Kraaijd V., & Garnefskid, N. **(2016)** Cognitive Emotion Regulation, Anxiety and Depression in Adults with Autism Spectrum Disorder. Research in Autism Spectrum Disorders, **22: 34-44**

Butler, R. C. & Gillis, J. M.(**2011**) The Impact of Labels and Behaviors on the Stigmatization of Adults with Asperger's Disorder. Journal of Autism and Developmental Disorders, **41(6): 741-749. DOI:10.1007/s10803-010-1093-9**

Byers, E. S. & Nichols, S. **(2014)** Sexual Satisfaction of High Functioning Adults with Autism Spectrum Disorder. Sexuality and Disability, **32(3): 365-382**

Carroll, M. R. & Wiggins, J. **(1990)** Elements of Group Counseling: Back to The Basics, Denver Colorado: Love Pub Duck, S. (1986) Human Relationships, London: Sage Pub

Eapen, V & Guan, J. **(2016)** Parental Quality of Life in Autism Spectrum Disorder: Current Status and Future Directions. Acta Psychoathol, **2:5DOI: 10.4172/2469-6676.100031**

Edmonds, G. & Worton, D. **(2006)** The Asperger Social Guide, London: Sage Pub

Edmonds, G. & Worton, D. **(2006**) The Asperger Personal Guide, London: Sage Pub

Engström, I., Ekström, L. & Emilsson, B. **(2003)** Psychological Functioning in a Group of Swedish Adults with Asperger Syndrome or High-Functioning Autism. Autism, **7(1): 99-110**

Fast, Y. et al. **(2004)** Employment for Individuals with Asperger Syndrome or Non-Verbal Learning Disability, London: Jessica Kingsley Pub

Freedman, S. **(2010)** Developing College Skills in Students with Autism and Asperger's Syndrome. London: Jessica Kingsley Publishers

Frith, U. (Ed.)(**1991)** Autism and Asperger Syndrome, UK: Cambridge University Press

Glass, L. Ph.D. **(2006)** I Know What You're Thinking (Hebrew translation)

Grandin T. & Duffy, K. **(2004)** Developing Talents Careers for Individuals with Asperger Syndrome and High Functioning Autism, Shawnee Mission KS: APC Publishing co.

Goleman, D. **(1995)** Emotional Intelligence, N.Y: Bantam Books

Goleman, D. **(2007)** Social Intelligence (Hebrew translation)

Goodyear, B. **(2008)** Coaching People with Asperger's Syndrome,.London: Karnac Books

Haadon, M. **(2004)** The Curious Incident of the Dog in the

Night-Time (Hebrew translation)

Henault, I. **(2005)** Asperger's Syndrome and Sexuality: From Adolescence through Adulthood. London: Jessica Kingsley Publishers

Hendrickx, S. & Newton, K. **(2007)** Asperger – A Love Story, London: Jessica Kingsley Pub

Hofvander, B. et al **(2009)** Psychiatric and Psychological Problems in Adults with Normal-Intelligence Autism Spectrum Disorder. BMC Psychiatry. **9 (35). DOI:10.1186/1471-244x-9-35**

Joselson, R. **(1996)** The Space Between Us, California: Sage Pub

Kapp, S. K., Gantman, A. & Laugeson, E. A. **(2011)** Transition to Adulthood for High-Functioning Individuals with Autism Spectrum Disorder. In M. R. Mohammadi (Ed.)(, A Comprehensive Book on Autism Spectrum Disorders(**pp. 451-478).** Croatia:In-Tech

Kraus, K. & Hulse-Killacky, D. **(1996)** Balancing Process and Content in Groups: A Metaphor. The Journal for Specialists in Group Work, (**21(2)**

Klin, A., Volkmar, F. R. & Sparrow, S. S.)Eds.( )2000(Asperger .Syndrome, N.Y: Guilford Press

Lever, A. G. & Geurts, H. M. **(2016)** Psychiatric Co-Occurring Symptoms and Disorders in Young, Middle-Aged, and Older Adults with Autism Spectrum Disorder. Journal of Autism and Developmental Disorders, **46, 1916-1930. DOI: 10.1007/ s10803016-2722-8**

Lovett J. P. **(2005)** Solutions for Adults with Asperger Syndrome,

Gloucester MA: Fair Wind Press

Marsack, C. (2016) An Examination of Quality of Life of Parents of Adult Children Diagnosed with Autism Spectrum Disorder. Wayne State University Dissertations. 1461https://digitalcommons. wayne.edu/oa_dissertations/1461

Merkler, E. E. (2007) The Experience of Isolation and Loneliness in Young Adults with High-Functioning Autism. University of North Carolina, PhD. Department of Psychology(Clinical Psychology) Chapel Hill: University of North Carolina

Meyer R.N. (2001) Asperger Syndrome Employment Workbook, London: Jessica Kingsley Pub

Miller, W. R. & Rollnick, S. (2012) Motivational Interviewing: Helping People Change (3rd ed.) New York: Guilford

Molcho, S. Körpersprache (Hebrew translation)

Moreno, S., Wheeler, M. & Parkinson, K. (2012) The Parent's Guide to Asperger Syndrome. London:Jessica Kingsley Publishers

Patrick N.J. (2008) Social Skills for Teenagers and Adults with Asperger Syndrome, London: Jessica Kingsley Pub

Prince-Hughes, D. (2006) Song of the Gorillas

Reber A. S. (1985) Dictionary of Psychology

Robison, J.E. (2007) Look Me in The Eye, N.Y: Crown Pub

Simsion, G. The Rosie Project (Hebrew translation)

Sinclair,J. (1992) Bridging the Gaps: An Inside-Out View pf Autism. In E. Schoplet & G. Mesibov (Eds.),High Fuctioning Individuals with Autism (pp.294-302). New York: Plenum

Slater-Walker G. & Christopher (2002) An Asperger Marriage, London: Jessica Kingsley Pub.

Stanford, A. (2006) Asperger Syndrome and Long TermRelationship, London: Jessica Kingsley Pub

Strunz, S. (2017) et al. Romantic Relationship and Relationship Satisfaction among Adults with Asperger Syndrome and High-Functioning Autism. Journal of Clinical Psychology, 73(1): 113.125

Szatmari, P. (2000) In Klin et al. Asperger Syndrome, N.Y: .Guilford Press

Tantam, D. (1991) Asperger Syndrome in Adulthood. In U. Frith (Ed), Autism and Asperger Syndrome (pp. 147-183). Cambridge, .UK: Cambridge University Press

Tantam, D. (2000) In Klin et al. Adolescence and Adulthood of Individuals with Asperger Syndrome, Modes of N.Y: Guildford Press

Trubanova, A. (2014) et al. Under-Identification of ASD in Females: A Case Series Illustrating the Unique Presentation of ASD in Young Adult Females. Scandinavian Journal of Child and Adolescent Psychiatry and Psychology, 2(2) 66-76

Van Bergeijk, E. et al. (2008) Supporting More Able Students on the Autism Spectrum: College and Beyond. Journal of Autism and Developmental Disorders, 38(7): 1359-1370. DOI: 10.1007/ s10803 007-0524-8

Van Bourgondien, M. E. (2014) et al. Families of Adults with Autism Spectrum Disorders. In F. R. Volkmar, B. Reichow & J.

McPartland (Eds.), Adolescents and Adults with Autism Spectrum Disorders **(pp. 15-40).** New York: Springer

Van der Horst, M. & Coffé, H. **(2012)** How Friendship Network Characteristics Influence Subjective Well-Being. Social Indicators .Research, **107(3): 509-529**

Wenzel, C. & Rowley, L**. (2010)** Teaching Social Skills and Academic Strategies to College Students with Asperger's Syndrome. [.Teaching Exceptional Children, **42(5): 44-50**

Whitehouse, A. J. **(2009)** et al. Friendship, Loneliness and Depression in Adolescents with Asperger's Syndrome. Journal of .Adolescence, **32(2): 309-322**

Whitaker, D. S. **(2001**) Using Groups to Help People (secondedition), London: Brunner-Routledge

Willey, L. H. **(1999)** Pretending to be Normal: Living with Asperger's Syndrome. Jessica Kingsley Publishers: London and Philadelphia

Willey, L. H. **(2001)** Asperger Syndrome in The Family, London: .Jessica Kingsley Pub

Wolf, L. E., Brown, J. T. & Bork, R. K. *(2009)* Students with Asperger Syndrome: A Guide for College Personnel. Shawnee .Mission, KS: Autism Asperger Pub. Co

Yalom, I. D. **(1995)** The Theory and Practice of Group Psychotherapy **(4th edition),** N.Y: Basic Books

Yurkiewicz, I. (2009) Overlooked and Under-Diagnosed: Distinct Expression of Asperger's Syndrome in Females. The Yale Review of Undergraduate Research in Psychology, 1)1(p: 80-91)